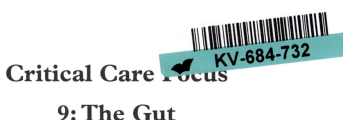

Critical Care Focus

9: The Gut

Critical Care Focus

9: The Gut

Books

© BMJ Books 2002
BMJ Books is an imprint of the BMJ Publishing Group

First published in 2002
by BMJ Books, BMA House, Tavistock Square,
London WC1H 9JR

www.bmjbooks.com
www.ics.ac.uk

British Library Cataloguing in Publication Data

A catalogue record for this book is available from the British Library

ISBN 0-7279-1679-3

Typeset by Newgen Imaging Systems (P) Ltd, Chennai.
Printed and bound in Spain by GraphyCems, Navarra

Contents

Critical Care Focus series

Also available:

Contributors

Anna M Batchelor
Consultant in Anaesthesia & Intensive Care Medicine, Royal Victoria Hospital, Newcastle-upon-Tyne, UK

Mark C Bellamy
Consultant in Anaesthesia & Intensive Care Medicine, St James University Hospital, Leeds, UK

John R Clark
Specialist Registrar in Anaesthesia, Sheffield School of Anaesthesia, Sheffield, UK

Jane Eddleston
Consultant in Anaesthesia & Intensive Care, Manchester Royal Infirmary, Manchester, UK

Helen F Galley
Senior Lecturer in Anaesthesia & Intensive Care, University of Aberdeen, Aberdeen, UK

Ulf Haglund
Professor of Surgery and Surgeon-in-Chief, Uppsala University Hospital, Uppsala, Sweden

John C Marshall
Professor of Surgery, University of Toronto, Toronto, Canada

Nigel Scott
Consultant Colorectal and Intestinal Failure Surgeon, Hope Hospital, Manchester, UK

Paul Winwood
Consultant in Gastroenterology, Royal Bournemouth Hospital, Bournemouth, UK

Preface to the Critical Care Focus series

The Critical Care Focus series aims to provide a snapshot of current thoughts and practice, by renowned experts. The complete series should provide a comprehensive guide for all health professionals on key issues in today's field of critical care. The volumes are deliberately concise and easy to read, designed to inform and provoke. Most chapters are produced from transcriptions of lectures given at the Intensive Care Society meetings and represent the views of world leaders in their fields.

Helen F Galley

Introduction

Gut dysfunction during enteral feeding

Anna M Batchelor

It is generally accepted that enteral feeding is preferable to parenteral feeding for critically ill patients, since it reduces mortality, it decreases the number of complications and of course it is much cheaper than parenteral nutrition. However, achieving targets for feeding remains problematic since delayed gastric emptying, common in such patients, can be a cause of feeding cessation. This article discusses the physiological mechanisms of delayed gastric emptying, the ways in which it can be assessed, and what can be done to remedy matters.

Diarrhoea

Mark C Bellamy

Diarrhoea in critically ill patients on the intensive care unit is an underestimated but common problem. In extreme cases, diarrhoea is endemic, and it can be a significant cause of death, particularly in places such as Asia, where specialised diarrhoea hospitals and even diarrhoea intensive care units have been established to deal with the problem. In Western hospitals, diarrhoea may result from critical illness directly, as a consequence of enteral feeding, antibiotic use or nosocomial infection. Some novel therapeutic approaches have suggested possibilities for the future.

Management of gastrointestinal fistulae

Nigel Scott

Post-operative gastrointestinal fistulae can arise due to gut injury from one of three possible mechanisms following abdominal surgery. The global management of the post-operative fistula patient can be summarised using the '4 Rs': Resuscitation, Restitution, Reconstruction and Rehabilitation. This article outlines the approach of the Intestinal Failure Unit at Hope Hospital, Manchester, UK, in dealing with intestinal fistulae. The large majority of patients referred to this unit are ultimately discharged home – only about 10% of those referred die after admission. The usual cause of death is multiple organ failure. Not surprisingly death is related to poor performance score, low serum albumin and age at referral. Older patients and patients with significant co-morbidity do particularly badly.

The gut as the motor of organ failure

John C Marshall

Data from a large number of published human studies support the hypothesis that the gastrointestinal tract contributes to morbidity and mortality in critically ill patients on the intensive care unit. Changes in proximal gut flora in the critically ill patient predict nosocomial infection with the same organism, while therapeutic measures targeting the gut clearly reduce rates of nosocomial infection and may have an impact on mortality. Modulation of the systemic inflammatory response through gut-derived measures has been no more successful than modulation of that response through more conventional systemic forms of mediator-directed therapy. But although the gastrointestinal tract is an important factor in nosocomial infection, to what extent does infection *per se* alter outcome in critical illness? The aim of this article is to provide a background to the evolution of the concept that in the critically ill patient the gut and its interactions with the liver play an important role in the clinical picture commonly seen in critically ill patients.

Mesenteric ischaemia

Ulf Hagland, Helen F Galley

In this article the physiology of the intestinal circulation of importance for the understanding of intestinal ischaemia is briefly outlined. The key to our understanding and successful treatment of intestinal ischaemia lies in a better knowledge of this physiology. The potential for intestinal vasoconstriction causing non-occlusive intestinal ischaemia is discussed, and the role of the reperfusion component of ischaemic injury. Maintenance of the mucosal cell barrier is essential in preventing the translocation of bacteria and endotoxin into the portal circulation and mesenteric lymphatics and the importance of this in the critically ill patient is addressed.

Medical management of non-variceal upper gastrointestinal haemorrhage

Paul Winwood

Acute upper gastrointestinal haemorrhage is a relatively common reason for admission to hospital and until recently there has been little change in mortality over the last fifty years. Acute bleeding also occurs in patients already in hospital and contributes significantly to overall mortality. Critically ill patients in particular are at increased risk of developing bleeding in the upper gastrointestinal tract, usually as a result of peptic ulceration. Most patients with acute haemorrhage are managed conservatively or with endoscopic intervention but some ultimately require surgery to arrest the haemorrhage. Endoscopic therapy has become a mainstay of the managing of upper gastrointestinal haemorrhage and this is the area where there has been perhaps the most advances in the last decade. This article describes the incidence and risk of re-bleeding and mortality in patients with bleeding ulcers, and describes available therapeutic options.

Acute pancreatitis

John R Clark, Jane Eddleston

Acute pancreatitis is a common disease on the intensive care unit, which is ruled by its complications, despite considerable increases in knowledge (as a result of animal studies) concerning the seminal events within the pancreatic acinar cell at the evolution of the acute inflammation. This article describes the epidemiology, aetiology and controversial clinical issues including feeding, new therapies and thoughts on future therapeutic options.

1: Gut dysfunction during enteral feeding

ANNA M BATCHELOR

Introduction

It is generally accepted that enteral feeding is preferable to parenteral feeding for critically ill patients, since it reduces mortality, it decreases the number of complications and of course it is much cheaper than parenteral nutrition (Box 1.1). However, achieving targets for feeding remains problematic since delayed gastric emptying, common in such patients, can be a cause of feeding cessation. This article discusses the physiological mechanisms of delayed gastric emptying, the ways in which it can be assessed, and what can be done to remedy matters.

Box 1.1 Reason to feed patients by the enteral route

- Preservation of gut mucosa
- Stimulation of host defence
- Prevention of bacterial translocation
- Improved anastomotic healing
- Preservation of beneficial gut bacteria
- Improved outcome
- Cost
- Safety

Problems with enteral feeding

Adam and Batson[1] reported the incidence of problems associated with enteral feeding in various groups of patients admitted to intensive care units (ICUs) in two district general and three university hospitals in the UK. All patients (n = 193) received enteral feeding for more than 24 hours and on average, only 76% of the quantity of feed prescribed was actually delivered to the patient. The two main problems preventing delivery of feed were gut dysfunction and planned stoppage for procedures. Those units with feeding protocols performed better in terms of feed delivery. Feeding was stopped completely in 11% of patients and in half of these this was due to gastric dysfunction. This study showed that problems with gut function and elective cessation of feeding prior to a procedure were the main causes of failure to feed to target. The authors recommended the use of well-defined feeding protocols since their use led to a greater volume of feed delivered.

In a similar study in the USA, by McClave *et al.*[2] the factors that impact on the delivery of enteral tube feeding were investigated in 44 medical ICU or coronary care unit patients who received only enteral tube feeding. It was found that only 78·1% of the feed volume prescribed was actually administered to the patient; in addition the prescribed volume was only 65·6% of goal requirements. Therefore these patients received on average only 51·6% of their nutritional requirements. Of the 24 patients who were able to be weighed more than half lost weight during enteral tube feeding. Enteral tube feeding was halted in 84% of patients and 66% of these stoppages were judged to be due to causes which could have been avoided. McClave and colleagues concluded that the way in which enteral tube feeding is delivered to ICU patients provides inadequate nutritional support partly due to underprescribing and inappropriate cessation of feed.

Box 1.2 Causes of delayed gastric emptying

- Diabetes mellitus
- Head injury
- Burns
- Laparotomy
- Pancreatitis
- Spinal cord injury
- Hyperglycaemia
- Hypokalaemia
- Opiates
- Anti-cholinergics
- Pain
- Sepsis

Slow gastric emptying

There are lots of reasons why gastric emptying is delayed (Box 1.2). Patients with diabetes often have a problem with gastric emptying due to autonomic neuropathy and hyperglycaemia, even in non-diabetics, interferes with the ability to empty the stomach. There are plenty of other causes of delayed gastric emptying. Perhaps the most irritating is that the use of opiates for pain relief will have the side effect of delaying gastric emptying, but the stress of inadequate pain relief also causes slow gastric emptying. Sepsis also results in slow gastric emptying, and this change may be one of the first signs of new sepsis in a previously successfully enterally fed patient.

Gastric physiology

The stomach functionally comprises two parts – the fundus, which acts as a reservoir and the antrum. Active relaxation of the stomach occurs in response to vagal or psychogenic stimulation and impulses from the mouth and oesophagus. Thus increases in gastric volume do not cause increases in pressure. The mainstay of measurements of gut motility is pressure monitoring, and this lack of pressure rise makes it difficult to measure proximal gastric function in the ICU. The proximal stomach, composed of the fundus and upper body, shows low frequency, sustained contractions responsible for generating a basal pressure within the stomach and propelling food into the gastric antrum.

The distal stomach, composed of the lower body and antrum, develops strong peristaltic waves of contraction which increase in amplitude as they propagate toward the pylorus. There is a pacemaker in the smooth muscle of the greater curvature that generates rhythmic slow waves from which action potentials and hence peristaltic contractions propagate. The pylorus is functionally part of this region of the stomach – when the peristaltic contraction reaches the pylorus, its lumen is effectively obliterated. The contractions generate a pressure gradient from the stomach to small intestine and chyme is thus delivered to the small intestine in spurts. Motility in both the proximal and distal regions of the stomach is controlled by a very complex set of neural and hormonal signals for example motilin, and neurotensin increase gastric emptying and secretin and catecholamines delay emptying. Nervous control originates from the enteric nervous system as well as parasympathetic (predominantly vagus nerve) and sympathetic systems. A large battery of hormones has been shown to influence gastric motility – for example, both gastrin and cholecystokinin act to relax the proximal stomach and enhance contractions in the distal stomach.

The principal determinants of the rate of gastric emptying are volume and composition. However, if the fluid is hypertonic or acidic or rich in nutrients such as fatty acids, the rate of gastric emptying will be considerably slower. Nutrient density is sensed predominantly in the small intestine by osmoreceptors and chemoreceptors, and relayed to the stomach as inhibitory neural and hormonal messages that delay emptying by altering the patterns of gastric motility. The presence of fat in the small intestine is the most potent inhibitor of gastric emptying, resulting in relaxation of the proximal stomach and diminished contractions of the distal stomach – when the fat has been absorbed, the inhibitory stimulus is removed and productive gastric motility resumes.

Intestinal physiology

The small intestine generates a wide variety of motor patterns to meet motility requirements in different situations. The small intestine produces a number of different contractions in various spatial and temporal patterns thus promoting efficient digestion, absorption, and propulsion of ingested material. Contractile activity of the small intestine is co-ordinated by an interplay of myogenic, neural (parasympathetic and sympathetic), and chemical controls. These contractions may cause mixing and agitation of luminal contents with slow distal propulsion. Occasionally, an individual contraction of large amplitude and long duration migrates over several centimetres and may rapidly propel the contents over this distance. All parts of the small bowel have an intrinsic frequency of motor activity; this is greatest in the duodenum which consequently acts as the pacemaker. Between meals, when digestion is complete, the small intestine generates migrating motor complexes.

Migrating motor complex

The migrating motor complex is a distinct pattern of electromechanical activity observed in gastrointestinal smooth muscle during fasting. It is thought to serve a "housekeeping" role and sweep residual undigested material through the gut. Phase 1 is a period of smooth muscle quiescence lasting 45 to 60 minutes, during which there are only rare action potentials and contractions. Phase 2 is a period of roughly 30 minutes of irregular contractile activity which progressively increases in frequency. Phase 3 is 5 to 15 minutes of regular powerful contractions, originating in the stomach and propagated through the small intestine. In contrast to the digestive period, the pylorus remains open during these peristaltic contractions, allowing many indigestible materials to pass into the small intestine.

An increase in gastric, biliary and pancreatic secretion is also seen in conjunction with the motor activity. These secretions probably aid in the cleansing activity of the migrating motor complex and assist in preventing a build-up of bacterial populations in the proximal segments of the digestive tube. Feeding abolishes a migrating motor complex and restores a digestive pattern of motility.

Critical illness and intestinal motility

Limited evidence has shown that migrating motor activity is frequently abnormal after surgery or in patients who are critically ill. Toumadre et al.[3] studied the effects of major abdominal surgery on small intestinal motility, and the motor complex patterns in critically ill patients in response to enteral feeding. A multi-lumen tube was used to monitor pressures at 12 points, distributed between the antrum and 100 cm distal to the pylorus in 11 patients undergoing aortic aneurysm repair. An additional lumen allowed enteral feeding into the duodenum. The study showed bursts of small intestinal pressure waves resembling phase 3 migrating motor activity in all patients immediately after surgery. During mechanical ventilation, the timing of bursts along the segment evaluated was frequently abnormal for phase 3 activity, although when patients were not being ventilated, the migration pattern of the bursts was more typical of phase 3 activity. A phase 2 pattern of pressure waves was not seen. More importantly, in the six patients who received enteral feeding, migrating motor activity was not abolished by feeding, contrary to normal phase 3 activity. The persistence of pressure wave bursts is likely to have implications for the delivery of enteral nutrition.

Bosscha and colleagues[4] determined gastrointestinal motility characteristics in relation to gastric retention in seven mechanically ventilated patients and nine healthy volunteers using antro-duodenal manometry, performed during fasting and gastric feeding. During the fasting state, under sedation with either midazolam or propofol and morphine, the migrating motor complex in patients was significantly shortened compared to healthy volunteers. During gastric tube feeding, the motility pattern did not convert to a normal post-prandial pattern until morphine was discontinued. A phase 3 pattern was seen during gastric tube feeding in most patients during morphine administration and most motor activity began in the duodenum rather than the gastric antrum during gastric feeding. Gastric retention during enteral feeding was correlated negatively with antral motor activity. These data suggest that morphine administration affects antro-duodenal motility in mechanically ventilated patients and that the motility patterns seen indicate that early administration of enteral feeding might be more effective into the duodenum or jejunum than into the stomach in such patients. Clearly being in the ICU receiving sedative medication, opiates and mechanical ventilation affects gastrointestinal motility.

Figure 1.1, also from the work of Bosscha,[4] shows the relationship of gastric residual volume and the motility index of the antrum – which takes into account both the number of antral contractions and the height of those

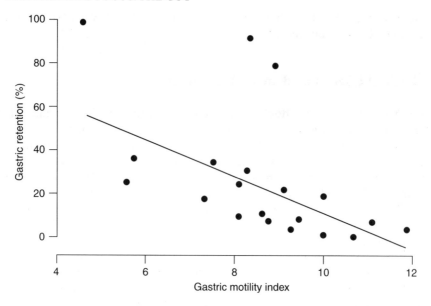

Figure 1.1 The relationship between gastric retention and antral motility index – which takes into account both the number of antrum contractions and the height of those contractions – in seven mechanically ventilated patients. Reproduced with permission from Bosscha K, et al. Crit Care Med 1998;26:1510–17.[4]

contractions. It can be seen that the greater the antrum motility index; i.e. the harder the antrum was working, the less likely was gastric retention. However, it should be remembered that both these studies are very small with only 11 and seven patients and not representative of the general ICU population.

There are also studies which have used the instillation of barium into different parts of the gastrointestinal tract during surgery as a model for what happens in critical illness. The movement of the barium can then be assessed – this work shows that if the barium is put into the stomach it takes a relatively long time to pass into the duodenum post-operatively, but if barium is put into the duodenum it will reach the terminal ileum within 24 hours, suggesting that after surgery the problem is gastric emptying rather than small bowel motility.

Assessment of gastric emptying

There are several techniques possible to assess gastric emptying (Box 1.3), but perhaps the gold standard is to use radiolabelled feed – scintigraphy. The non-invasive ^{13}C-octanoic acid breath test to measure gastric emptying in ventilated critically ill patients was recently reported in *Critical Care Medicine*.[5] Thirty unselected, mechanically ventilated, critically ill patients

---

Box 1.3 Techniques to assess gastric emptying

- Scintigraphy
- ^{13}C-octanoic acid breath test
- Paracetamol absorption
- Gastric residual volume
- Bowel sounds

---

receiving gastric feeding and 22 healthy volunteers were studied. Following intra-gastric infusion of 100 ml of enteral feed (Ensure) labelled with ^{13}C-octanoic acid in patients, end-expiratory breath samples were collected from the ventilator circuit. Breath samples were also collected from supine volunteers after an identical nasogastric infusion. Breath $^{13}CO_2$ was measured by isotope ratio mass spectrometry. Importantly, the breath test did not interfere with patient care. The labelled carbon dioxide level was >1% in 99·8% of breath samples, indicating satisfactory end-expiratory timing. The study revealed that gastric emptying was slower in patients compared with volunteers and the authors concluded that the ^{13}C-octanoic acid breath test is a novel and useful bedside technique to measure gastric emptying in critically ill patients.

Paracetamol is absorbed in the duodenum and there have been several studies using the absorption of this drug as a way of assessing the effects of other drugs on gastric emptying.[6,7] There are some problems with the use of this technique. The area under the curve of the paracetamol level can be affected by factors other than the rate of gastric emptying and delivery of paracetamol from the stomach into the duodenum. The rate of metabolism, the rate of elimination, and the volume of distribution are all important. Some studies have looked much more in detail at pharmokinetic profiling of paracetamol to try to eliminate the other components which might affect paracetamol level, unrelated to the amount of gastric emptying.

Gastric residual volume has been used to assess gastric emptying, mainly because it is possible, despite the fact that it is incredibly inaccurate. Almost 10 years ago, McClave[8] reported a study to determine the residual volume which indicated intolerance or inadequate gastric emptying. The residual volume correlated poorly with physical examination and radiography findings. Twenty healthy normal volunteers, eight stable patients with gastrostomy tubes *in situ*, and 10 critically ill patients were studied for eight hours while receiving enteral feeding. Some patients had residual volumes above 150 ml, but so did some healthy volunteers. Two hundred ml was the least residual volume that would have allowed continuation of feeding in the normal volunteers and has thus been adopted as the amount of aspirate indicating tolerance during enteral feeding.

Finally, the presence or absence of bowel sounds bears no relationship whatsoever as to whether patients will tolerate feeding.

Improving gastric emptying

There are two options for managing the problem of the impaired gastric emptying in critically ill patients: the first is to use pro-kinetic agents and the second is to put the feed further down the intestinal tract. Pro-kinetic agents include metoclopramide, erthyromycin and cisapride; the latter of course has unfortunately been withdrawn from use.

Pro-kinetic agents

Metoclopromide is a dopamine2 receptor antagonist which enhances cholinergic induced peristalsis. MacLaren et al.[9] recently investigated the comparative efficacy of enteral cisapride, metoclopramide, erythromycin, and placebo for promoting gastric emptying in 20 critically ill patients with intolerance to gastric enteral feeding. Patients received 10 mg cisapride, 200 mg erythromycin ethylsuccinate, 10 mg of metoclopramide, or placebo every 12 hours for two days. Paracetamol was also given to quantify gastric emptying. These workers concluded that single enteral doses of metoclopramide or cisapride are equally effective for improving gastric emptying in critically ill patients but metoclopramide may also provide a quicker onset.

It has been known for a number of years that erythromycin improves diabetic-related problems in gastric emptying and probably works as a motilin agonist. It accelerates gastric emptying in diabetic patients and increases phase 3 antral motility in a dose dependent manner, at levels below those required for bacterial killing. Otterson and Sarna[10] studied the small intestinal motor effects of oral and intravenous erythromycin in dogs. After control recordings with placebo, oral or intravenous erythromycin was given at 40% of the migrating motor complex cycle. Recordings were made after administration until normal contractile activity had returned or 12 hours post-drug administration. Low doses of erythromycin were found to initiate premature motor complex cycling. Erythromycin at high doses, however, prolonged the phase 3 cycle length and reduced the propagation velocity at all doses. Erythromycin also increased the incidence of retrograde giant contractions and vomiting. The findings suggest that erythromycin has multiple motor effects on the stomach and small intestine. Erythromycin may therefore aid gastric emptying but it can do it in one of two ways – up or down!

The effect of intravenous erythromycin on gastric emptying and the success of enteral feeding has also been reported in mechanically ventilated, critically ill patients with large gastric residual volumes (Figure 1.2).[11] Nasogastric feeding was successful in 9 of 10 patients treated with erythromycin and 5 of 10 who received placebo, suggesting that a single small dose of intravenous erythromycin may allow continuation of feeding in the short term.

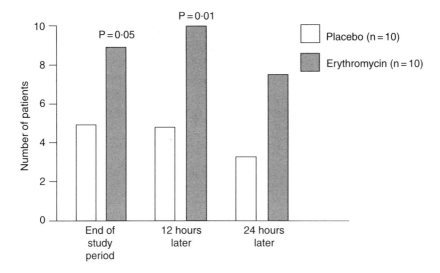

Figure 1.2 The effects of intravenous erythromycin therapy on successful enteral feeding. Reproduced with permission from Chapman MJ, et al. Crit Care Med 2000;28:2334–7.[11]

Jejunal tubes

Transpyloric small intestine feeding tube placement can be both difficult and tedious. All currently accepted techniques are associated with disadvantages and risk. There are a few ways in which feeding tubes can be introduced into the duodenum, including passive transport from the stomach and there are several studies, all of which show different rates of success, and may include pro-kinetic agents. The end of the tubes can also be weighted to aid transit. Zaloga[12] claims successful post-pyloric tube placement at the bedside in 92% of cases, a feat which few can reproduce.

Imaging-assisted placement is more consistently successful and is very safe but requires transfer of patients to the x ray department and this may require half an hour of screening which results in a large amount of time and radiation exposure. Blind manual bedside method for placing feeding tubes into the small bowel was compared with an ultrasound assisted bedside technique in 35 critically ill patients.[13] All patients were haemodynamically stable, mechanically ventilated, and required tube placement for short-term enteral feeding due to impaired gastric emptying. Blind, manual post-pyloric tube placement was always attempted first in all cases and successful placement was confirmed by x ray film. If after 30 min the tube did not enter the small bowel, a sonographic bedside technique was used. The blind manual method was successful in only 25·7% of patients. The average time for placement of the feeding tubes with this manual technique was 13·9 min. The ultrasound technique was successful in 84·6% of the remaining patients and the average time for placement 18·3 min.

Much more commonly, and definitely more successful if the expertise is available, is to use the Seldinger technique of endoscopic tube placement.

Grathwohl and colleagues[14] described bedside videoscopic placement using a fibreoptic scope through the feeding tube, in healthy volunteers and critically ill patients. Standard feeding tubes were placed under direct vision using a 2·2 mm fibreoptic scope through the feeding tube. Enteric structures were clearly seen through the feeding tube in all subjects and patients and the feeding tube could be advanced through the pylorus and into the duodenum based on visual landmarks in all individuals. Transpyloric tube placement was confirmed videoscopically and radiographically. This new technique obviously has the potential for rapid, accurate and safe feeding tube placement in patients requiring nutritional support.

Patient position

The prone position can be effective in mechanically ventilated patients to improve oxygenation but this position may affect gastric emptying and the ability to continue enteral feeding. However, Van der Voort[15] determined the tolerance of enteral feeding in enterally fed patients during supine and prone positions and found little difference in gastric residual volume between positions. The authors suggested that patients with a clinically significant gastric residual volume in one position are likely to have a clinically significant gastric residual volume in the other position.

Summary

In summary, my personal approach to the problem of delayed gastric emptying is as follows: have a feeding protocol which is adhered to by all members of the department. Patients should be sedated as little as possible, and opiates should be avoided. Avoid placing patients in the supine position and instead nurse them in an upright or semi-recumbent position. Pro-kinetic agents may be of use and I tend to use erythromycin if 24 hours of metoclopromide is unsuccessful. Jejunal tube placement may be required and any doubt in the ability of a patient to tolerate feeding should prompt early placement of these tubes to avoid longer periods of potential malnutrition. Perseverance is important, since although many patients may appear not to tolerate feeding, continued feeding with repeated attempts to increase the volumes administered will often succeed.

References

1   Adam S, Batson S. A study of problems associated with the delivery of enteral feed in critically ill patients in five ICUs in the UK. *Intensive Care Med* 1997; **23**:261–6.

2   McClave SA, Sexton LK, Spain DA, *et al.* Enteral tube feeding in the intensive care unit: factors impeding adequate delivery. *Crit Care Med* 1999;**27**:1252–6.

3   Toumadre JP, Barclay M, Fraser R, *et al.* Small intestinal motor patterns in critically ill patients after major abdominal surgery. *Am J Gastroenterol* 2001; **96**:2418–26.

4   Bosscha K, Nieuwenhuijs VB, Vos A, Samsom M, Roelofs JM, Akkermans LM. Gastrointestinal motility and gastric tube feeding in mechanically ventilated patients. *Crit Care Med* 1998;**26**:1510–17.

5   Toumadre JP, Davidson G, Dent J. Delayed gastric emptying in ventilated critically ill patients: Measurement by ^{13}C-octanoic acid breath test. *Crit Care Med* 2001;**29**:1744–9.

6   Cohen J, Aharon A, Singer P. The paracetamol absorption test: a useful addition to the enteral nutrition algorithm? *Clin Nutr* 2000;**19**(4):233–6.

7   Heyland DK, Tougas G, King D, Cook DJ. Impaired gastric emptying in mechanically ventilated, critically ill patients. *Intensive Care Med* 1996;**22**(12):1339–44.

8   McClave SA, Snider HL, Lowen CC, *et al.* Use of residual volume as a marker for enteral feeding intolerance: prospective blinded comparison with physical examination and radiographic findings. *J Parenter Enteral Nutr* 1992;**16**:99–105.

9   MacLaren R, Kuhl DA, Gervasio JM, *et al.* Sequential single doses of cisapride, erythromycin, and metoclopramide in critically ill patients intolerant to enteral nutrition: a randomized, placebo-controlled, crossover study. *Crit Care Med* 2000;**28**:438–44.

10 Otterson MF, Sarna SK. Gastrointestinal motor effects of erythromycin. *Am J Physiol* 1990;**259**:G355–63.

11 Chapman MJ, Fraser RJ, Kluger MT, Buist MD, De Nichilo DJ. Erythromycin improves gastric emptying in critically ill patients intolerant of nasogastric feeding. *Crit Care Med* 2000;**28**:2334–7.

12 Zaloga GP, Roberts PR. Bedside placement of enteral feeding tubes in the intensive care unit. *Crit Care Med* 1998;**26**:987–8.

13 Hernandez-Socorro CR, Marin J, Ruiz-Santana S, Santana L, Manzano JL. Bedside sonographic-guided versus blind nasoenteric feeding tube placement in critically ill patients. *Crit Care Med* 1996;**24**:1690–4.

14 Grathwohl KW, Gibbons RV, Dillard TA, *et al.* Bedside videoscopic placement of feeding tubes: development of fiberoptics through the tube. *Crit Care Med* 1997;**25**:629–34.

15 Van der Voort PH, Zandstra DF. Enteral feeding in the critically ill: comparison between the supine and prone positions: a prospective crossover study in mechanically ventilated patients. *Crit Care* 2001;**5**:216–20.

2: Diarrhoea

MARK C BELLAMY

Introduction

Diarrhoea in critically ill patients on the intensive care unit (ICU) is an underestimated but common problem. In extreme cases, diarrhoea is endemic, and it can be a significant cause of death, particularly in places such as Asia, where specialised diarrhoea hospitals and even diarrhoea ICUs have been established to deal with the problem. In Western hospitals, diarrhoea may result from critical illness directly, as a consequence of enteral feeding, antibiotic use or nosocomial infection.

Definition of diarrhoea

The first problem in addressing the issue of diarrhoea in the ICU is that even the definition of diarrhoea is inconsistent. There are relatively few papers in the literature which deal with diarrhoea in the ICU and even fewer which subscribe to a clear definition of what diarrhoea actually means. The definition in the *Shorter Oxford Dictionary* identifies diarrhoea as a disorder consisting of "the too frequent evacuation of too fluid faeces sometimes attended with griping pains". Of course such a definition is not terribly useful in the context of intensive care. In a study from the Veteran Administration Medical Center, the frequency and consistency of stools of all patients who were tube-fed during a three-month period were recorded prospectively and analysed in terms of eight definitions of diarrhoea derived from the literature. The extent of diarrhoea, reported as incidence and as percentage of days with diarrhoea, was used to determine differences among the definitions. The relationship between the extent of diarrhoea and duration of monitoring patients was also determined. Data from 29 patients monitored for a median of 13 days indicated that the definition of diarrhoea significantly influenced the reported incidence of, and percentage of days with, diarrhoea. Duration of monitoring showed a significant, positive relationship to the incidence of diarrhoea (i.e., the longer the duration, the more likely that diarrhoea was observed). When diarrhoea was reported as the percentage of days with diarrhoea, the influence of monitoring duration virtually disappeared.[1]

Although there are no clear definitions, most studies have criteria which use frequency and consistency to produce some sort of scoring system. A study by Guenter and Sweed[2] addressed the problem of quantifying diarrhoea in enterally fed patients. A major problem in determining whether diarrhoea exists in enterally fed patients is the quantification of stool output. On the basis of this need, Guenter and Sweed developed a stool output assessment tool, which they tested for validity and reliability. Reliability and validity were determined by using staff nurses' and principal investigators' observations. Observers rated the bowel movement on size and consistency and on whether the movement was thought to represent "diarrhoea". Unfortunately this useful scoring system has not been used in other studies.

Spectrum of diarrhoea

Diarrhoea in the intensive care unit is a spectrum of conditions ranging from something which is mildly inconvenient to clinicians, to a major systemic disturbance, with an inherent mortality. In some parts of the world, dedicated diarrhoea hospitals exist to deal with the catastrophic electrolyte disturbance caused by severe diarrhoea. In places such as Egypt or India, diarrhoea hospitals and even diarrhoea intensive care units are established in the major centres. We have all seen pictures of cholera victims in Bangladesh, where the severity of illness and the degree of systemic disturbance is clear and we can therefore understand why it is necessary to have major units to deal with the problem.

To identify risk factors for death among children with diarrhoea, Mitra and colleagues investigated a cohort of 496 children, aged less than 5 years, admitted to the ICU of a diarrhoeal disease hospital in Bangladesh.[3] Clinical and laboratory records of children who died and of those who recovered in the hospital were compared. Deaths were significantly higher among those who had altered consciousness, hypoglycaemia, septicaemia, paralytic ileus, toxic colitis, necrotizing enterocolitis, haemolytic-uraemic syndrome, invasive or persistent diarrhoea, dehydration, electrolyte imbalances, and malnutrition. The risk of death in girls was twice as high as for boys. Girls with severe infections were brought to the hospital less often than boys and the time lapse between onset of symptoms and hospital admission was significantly higher in female children than male. Despite the dedicated hospitals, in a recent study of causes of child death in Bangladesh, Baqu et al. showed that deaths from diarrhoea have decreased little.[4]

Causes of diarrhoea

It is well recognised that diarrhoea is an important problem in critically ill patients and in some parts of the world it is a frequent cause of death, but diarrhoea is not necessarily a trivial problem in ICU in this country. In Western practice diarrhoea usually results from nosocomial infection, from critical illness per se, that is gut dysfunction, or it may be a complication of feeding or antibiotic usage.

Many studies have linked diarrhoea with enteral feeding although it is not a universally supported view and relatively few studies have looked at diarrhoea as a primary end point, but have looked at feeding complications in general. Levinson and Bryce undertook a relatively small prospective study to determine whether there is any relationship between enteral feeding, gastric colonisation and diarrhoea in critically ill patients.[5] Sixty-two critically ill patients from an intensive care unit of a major teaching hospital, who satisfied the usual criteria for enteral feeding, were randomised to receive enteral feeding or not, for three days followed by a second randomisation to enteral feeding or not for a further three days. Diarrhoea was recorded and cultures taken of both gastric aspirates and stool. The results revealed no significant difference in the incidence of diarrhoea whether patients were enterally fed or not. Gastric colonisation was also unrelated to feeding practice and to the development of diarrhoea. The authors concluded that in the critically ill patient, enteral feeding does not cause or promote diarrhoea. However, it should be noted that this was a small study, of only 62 patients, over a very short study period.

Larger feeding studies have not necessarily used diarrhoea as a primary end point. Adam and Batson[6] published a study in *Intensive Care Medicine* which described the incidence of problems associated with enteral feeding in different patient groups and ICUs. They compared this incidence with specific feeding protocols and volumes of feed delivered, with the intention of identifying future study interventions likely to improve delivery of enteral feed and to manage or eliminate problems. They studied 193 patients who received enteral feeding for 24 hours, for a total of 1929 patient-days. On average, only 76% of the quantity of feed prescribed was delivered to the patient. The two main problems preventing delivery of feed were gut dysfunction and elective stoppage for procedures. ICUs with well-defined feeding protocols delivered significantly greater volumes of feed than those without a protocol. Feeding was abandoned in 11% of patients, half of these due to gastric dysfunction. Only two of 193 patients were fed jejunally. The authors concluded that problems with gut function and stopping feed prior to a procedure were the major factors associated with the interruption in delivery of feed. In this study diarrhoea was a relatively minor factor and only about 18% of patients had significant diarrhoea and that was not the main reason for discontinuing feeding.

A big Spanish multi-centre study by Montejo was published on behalf of the Nutritional and Metabolic Working Group of the Spanish Society of Intensive Care Medicine and Coronary Units.[7] The frequency of gastrointestinal complications in a prospective cohort of critically ill patients receiving enteral nutrition and the effects on nutrient administration and the relationship to outcome was evaluated. A prospective cohort of 400 consecutive patients admitted to 37 multidisciplinary ICUs in Spain and receiving enteral nutrition was studied. Enteral, nutrition-related, gastrointestinal complications and their management were defined by consensus before data collection. During the one month study period a total of 3 778 enteral feeding days were analysed in 400 patients. The mean duration of enteral nutrition was 9·6 days. Mean elapsed time from ICU admission to the start of enteral feeding was 3·1 days; 66·2% of patients received a standard polymeric formula, and 33·8% received a disease-specific formula, administered mainly through a nasogastric tube. At least one gastrointestinal complication occurred in 251 patients (62·8%) during the feeding course, including: high gastric residuals, 39%; constipation, 15·7%; diarrhoea, 14·7%; abdominal distension, 13·2%; vomiting, 12·2%; and regurgitation, 5·5%. Enteral nutrition withdrawal as a consequence occurred in 15·2% of patients. The volume ratio (expressed as the ratio between administered and prescribed volumes of feed) was calculated daily and was used as an index of diet administration efficacy. Patients with gastric complications had a lower volume ratio, a longer length of stay, and higher mortality (31% vs. 16·1%). This study showed that the frequency of enteral nutrition-related gastric complications in critically ill patients is high, resulting in decreased nutrient. Enteral feeding, gastrointestinal intolerance also seems to prolong ICU stay and increase mortality. The mean time for ICU admission to enteral feeding was three days in this study and this may well be significant because as is well known, in most of the feeding studies on immunonutrition, the benefits are clearer where feeding is introduced earlier (see *Critical Care Focus Volume 7*[8]) and there are some studies which claim the benefit is seen only where feeding is introduced before three days. Overall, however, only 15% of all the patients, including those with diarrhoea, had to have their feeding stopped because of uncontrollable complications.

Antibiotic usage may also contribute to diarrhoea in acutely ill patients. Guenter and co-workers[9] studied the contribution of antibiotics to diarrhoea, and the benefit of fibre in patients on enteral feeding. One hundred patients were prospectively assigned either a fibre-free formula or a fibre-supplemented formula. Diarrhoea was defined as three or more loose or watery stools per day and occurred in 30% of all patients. Diarrhoea developed in 29 of the 71 patients who received antibiotics during, or within 2 weeks prior to, the feeding period, whereas only one of the 29 patients not receiving antibiotics developed diarrhoea. Among the 30 patients with diarrhoea, stool *Clostridium difficile* toxin was positive in a significant proportion. In this patient population, antibiotic usage was the factor most strongly associated with diarrhoea during tube feedings.

Nosocomial diarrhoeas are an important problem in hospitals,[10] and in critical care units in particular. Infectious causes of nosocomial diarrhoea are due to enteric pathogens in outbreak situations and virtually all of the causes are due to *Clostridium difficile*. *C. difficile* is a resident of the human colon and does not cause disease if its toxins are not elaborated. Chemotherapeutic agents, and more commonly, antibiotics, induce the elaboration of toxin A and B from *C. difficile* in the distal gastrointestinal tract. The spectrum of disease of *C. difficile* in hospitalized patients includes asymptomatic carriage to mild watery diarrhoea, fulminant and severe diarrhoea, and pseudomembranous enterocolitis. The treatment of *C. difficile* diarrhoea is usually with oral metronidazole or vancomycin, and *C. difficile* colitis is treated with intravenous metronidazole. Infection control measures are necessary to prevent the spread of this spore-forming organism within the institution since it is capable of surviving in the hospital environment for prolonged periods.

Perhaps the most important risk factor for transmission of *C. difficile* is physical proximity to other affected patients, i.e. space in the ICU and the use of side rooms to isolate infected patients. To examine physical proximity as a risk factor for the nosocomial acquisition of *C. difficile*- and antibiotic-associated diarrhoea Chang and Nelson[11] assessed a retrospective cohort of 2 859 patients admitted to a community hospital over a period of six months. Of these patients, 68 had nosocomial *C. difficile*-associated diarrhoea, and 54 had nosocomial antibiotic-associated diarrhoea. Significant risk factors for diarrhoea were, physical proximity to a patient with *C. difficile* infection, exposure to clindamycin, and the number of antibiotics taken. Thus a strict antibiotic policy such that certain antibiotics such as clindomycin, are restricted in their use, and remedial measures related to strict environmental controls, are important.

Prevention of diarrhoea

A number of novel approaches have been introduced recently to the problem of tube-fed associated diarrhoea. For some reason it has attracted great interest and novel therapeutic strategies have been introduced. The principal risk factors for tube-fed patients, include the things you would imagine, malnutrition, hypolabuminaemia, infection, previous failure of oral feeding regimens.

Saccharomyces boulardii is a thermophilic, non-pathogenic yeast administered for the prevention and treatment of a variety of diarrhoeal diseases.[12] However, the mechanisms by which *S. boulardii* controls diarrhoea remain elusive. The efficacy of this yeast has been attributed to several of its properties, such as its effect on the mucosa leading to an increase in disaccharidase activity or stimulation of the immune response. In animals, administration of *S. boulardii* provides protection against intestinal lesions caused by several diarrhoeal pathogens. *In vitro* studies have demonstrated that *S. boulardii* exerts antagonistic activity against various bacterial pathogens and studies have reported the adhesion of the *Salmonella enterica serovars Typhimurium* and *Enteritis* and of enteropathogenic *Escherichia coli* and enterohaemorrhagic *E. coli* to *S. boulardii*. A study designed to investigate the effect of this yeast on enteropathogenic *Escherichia coli*-associated disease demonstrated that *S. boulardii* abrogated several effects of *E. coli* on T84 cells, including delayed apoptosis of epithelial cells. The yeast did not modify the number of adherent bacteria but lowered by 50% the number of intracellular bacteria. Altogether, this study demonstrated that *S. boulardii* exerts a protective effect on epithelial cells after an enteropathogenic *Escherichia coli* adhesion by modulating the signalling pathway induced by bacterial infection.[13]

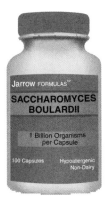

Figure 2.1 Commercially available Saccharomyces boulardii *preparation containing one billion organisms per capsule.*

S. boulardii has been used in several conditions, including pseudomembranous colitis, Crohn's disease, and immuno-suppressive diarrhoeas, for example in HIV and AIDS, although there are few randomised controlled clinical trials data in that setting (Figure 2.1). A study in ICU patients was reported by Bleichner and colleagues,[14] who assessed the preventive effect of *S. boulardii* on diarrhoea in critically ill, enterally fed patients and evaluated the risk factors for diarrhoea. Critically ill patients (n=128) whose need for enteral nutrition was expected to exceed six days, were studied in 11 intensive care units in teaching and general hospitals. Patients received either 500 mg *S. boulardii* four times a day or placebo. Diarrhoea was defined using a semi-quantitative score based on the volume and consistency of stools. Treatment with *S. boulardii* reduced the mean percentage of days with diarrhoea (Figure 2.2). In the control group, nine risk factors were significantly associated with diarrhoea, including non-sterile administration of nutrients in open containers, previous suspension of oral feeding, malnutrition, hypoalbuminaemia, sepsis syndrome, multiple organ failure, presence of an infection site, fever or hypothermia, and use of antibiotics. Five independent factors were associated with diarrhoea in a multivariate analysis: fever or hypothermia, malnutrition, hypoalbuminaemia, previous suspension of oral feeding, and presence of an infection site. After adjustment for these factors, the preventive effect of *S. boulardii* on diarrhoea was even more significant. This study therefore showed that *S. boulardii* treatment prevents diarrhoea in critically ill tube-fed patients, especially in patients at higher risk for diarrhoea. It is not yet known, however whether treatments of this type improve overall survival.

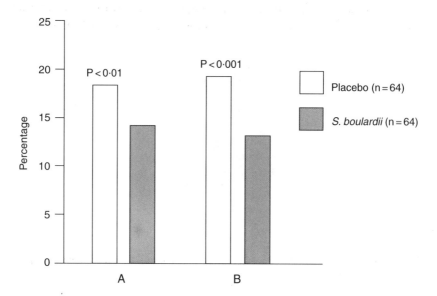

Figure 2.2 The effect of Saccharomyces boulardii *in critically ill enterally fed patients in terms of A. the percentage of days with diarrhoea in terms of feeding days and B. the percentage of days with diarrhoea in terms of observation days. Redrawn from data presented in Bleichner G, et al.* Intensive Care Med *1997;23:517-23.*[14]

Attempts to control enteral nutrition associated diarrhoea in the critically ill tube-fed patient by implementing feeding formulas enriched with fibre have not generally been successful. However, it was shown that enteral feeding containing soluble partially hydrolysed guar decreased the incidence of diarrhoea in a cohort of non-critically ill medicosurgical patients. Spapen *et al.* investigated whether this type of enteral feed could also influence stool production in patients with severe sepsis.[15] Patients with severe sepsis and septic shock were consecutively enrolled (n=25) and received either an enteral formula supplemented with 22 g/l partially hydrolysed guar or an isocaloric isonitrogenous control feed without fibre. Enteral feeding was provided through a nasogastric tube for a minimum of six days. A semi-quantitative score based on stool volume and consistency was used for daily assessment of diarrhoea. The mean frequency of diarrhoea days was significantly lower in patients receiving fibre than in those who did not. This recent study certainly suggested that total enteral nutrition supplemented with soluble fibre is beneficial in reducing the incidence of diarrhoea in enterally fed septic patients.

Conclusion

Diarrhoea can be a major cause of ICU admission in some parts of the world and has an inherent mortality. It can also occur as a consequence of ICU therapy (enteral feeding), nosocomial infection and antibiotic usage. Some novel therapeutic approaches have suggested possibilities for the future.

References

1   Bliss DZ, Guenter PA, Settle RG. Defining and reporting diarrhea in tube-fed patients – what a mess! *Am J Clin Nutr* 1992;**55**:753–9.
2   Guenter PA, Sweed MR. A valid and reliable tool to quantify stool output in tube-fed patients. *J Parenter Enteral Nutr* 1998;**22**:147–51.
3   Mitra AK, Rahman MM, Fuchs GJ. Risk factors and gender differentials for death among children hospitalized with diarrhoea in Bangladesh. *J Health Popul Nutr* 2000;**18**:151–6.
4   Baqu AH, Sabir AA, Begum N, Arifeen SE, Mitra SN, Black RE. Causes of childhood deaths in Bangladesh: an update. *Acta Paediatr* 2001;**90**:682–90.
5   Levinson M, Bryce A. Enteral feeding, gastric colonisation and diarrhoea in the critically ill patient: is there a relationship? *Anaesth Intensive Care* 1993;**21**:85–8.
6   Adam S, Batson S. A study of problems associated with the delivery of enteral feed in critically ill patients in five ICUs in the UK. *Intensive Care Med* 1997;**23**:261–6.
7   Montejo JC. Enteral nutrition-related gastrointestinal complications in critically ill patients: a multicenter study. The Nutritional and Metabolic Working Group of the Spanish Society of Intensive Care Medicine and Coronary Units. *Crit Care Med* 1999;**27**:1447–53.
8   Galley HF, ed. *Critical Care Focus, Volume 5: Antibiotic Resistance and Infection Control.* London: BMJ Books/Intensive Care Society, 2001.
9   Guenter PA, Settle RG, Perlmutter S, Marino PL, DeSimone GA, Rolandelli RH. Tube feeding-related diarrhea in acutely ill patients. *J Parenter Enteral Nutr* 1991;**15**:277–80.
10 Cunha BA. Nosocomial diarrhea. *Crit Care Clin* 1998;**14**:329–38.
11 Chang VT, Nelson K. The role of physical proximity in nosocomial diarrhea. *Clin Infect Dis* 2000;**31**:717–22.
12 Marteau PR, de Vrese M, Cellier CJ, Schrezenmeir J. Protection from gastrointestinal diseases with the use of probiotics. *Am J Clin Nutr* 2001;**73**:430S–6S.

13 Czerucka D, Dahan S, Mograbi B, Rossi B, Rampal P. *Saccharomyces boulardii* preserves the barrier function and modulates the signal transduction pathway induced in enteropathogenic *Escherichia coli*-infected T84 cells. *Infect Immun* 2000;**68**:5998–6004.

14 Bleichner G, Blehaut H, Mentec H, Moyse D. *Saccharomyces boulardii* prevents diarrhea in critically ill tube-fed patients. A multicenter, randomized, double-blind placebo-controlled trial. *Intensive Care Med* 1997;**23**:517–23.

15 Spapen H, Diltoer M, Van Malderen C, Opdenacker G, Suys E, Huyghens L. Soluble fiber reduces the incidence of diarrhoea in septic patients receiving total enteral nutrition: a prospective, double-blind, randomized, and controlled trial. *Clin Nutr* 2001;**20**:301–5.

3: Management of gastrointestinal fistulae

NIGEL SCOTT

Introduction

Post-operative gastrointestinal fistulae can arise due to gut injury from one of three possible mechanisms following abdominal surgery (Box 3.1). The global management of the post-operative fistula patient can be summarised using the "4 Rs": Resuscitation, Restitution, Reconstruction and Rehabilitation. This article outlines the approach of the Intestinal Failure Unit at Hope Hospital, Manchester, UK, in dealing with intestinal fistulae.[1,2]

Box 3.1   Causes of post-operative fistulae

- Unrecognised intestinal injury
- Breakdown of serotomy repair
- Breakdown of anastomosis

Resuscitation

Septic patients with multiple organ failure require immediate assessment and support of the airway, breathing and circulation, with patient transfer to a surgical high dependency unit (HDU) or the intensive care unit (ICU) for monitoring and/or organ support, if indicated. Large losses of gastrointestinal fluid directly equates with large losses of saline, since the enteric fluid sodium content is approximately 110 mmol/l; saline fluid resuscitation is therefore commonly required. Discharge of corrosive enteric enzymes and bile salts produces skin destruction, and protection of the skin and collection of these losses requires time-consuming and dedicated nursing resources. In addition, the morale of the patient and relatives, and also staff morale requires a form of "resuscitation" – if the fistula becomes a difficult and long term problem.

Restitution

Restitution is the restoration of the patient's biology to a situation where either spontaneous closure of the fistula can take place or it is reasonable to carry out surgical correction of the fistula. Thus, after the immediate assessment and resuscitation of the post-operative fistula patient, the next stage is to restore him or her to a state from which fistula closure – spontaneous or surgical – can take place. This requires attention to the acronym "SNAP" which stands for Sepsis, Nutrition, Anatomy and Plan.

SNAP

Sepsis

In the post-operative fistula patient, failure to contain and arrest the progress of intra-abdominal sepsis leads to continuation of multiple organ failure, ineffective nutritional support due to continued catabolism, and failure of fistula healing leading ultimately to the patient's death. Effective elimination of intra-abdominal sepsis is therefore mandatory and all patients with a post-operative fistula should undergo computed tomography (CT) evaluation of the abdomen for abscess formation as their baseline assessment. CT guided drainage is effective in managing isolated abscess collections contributing to the focus of sepsis. However, CT drainage is not successful if the collection is being directly fed by the fistulating gut. The more common situation is where the abscess and fistula are still connected within the abdominal cavity and a surgical strategy to exteriorise the gut must be undertaken (Figure 3.1). There are three basic surgical strategies to be considered to control intra-abdominal sepsis in these circumstances (Box 3.2).

The simplest strategy is to undertake a midline laparotomy, resect the fistula and exteriorise the two ends (Figure 3.1A). A procedure which is used less often but is useful if the patient has a "battle scarred" abdomen, involves going into the left quadrant and performing a very high jejunostomy (Figure 3.1B). This is a reasonably easy way to defunction fistulae, but it means that the patient is condemned to a period of parenteral nutrition.

Box 3.2   Surgical strategies to control intra-abdominal sepsis

- Resect enteric injury, exteriorise the ends
- Left upper quadrant laparotomy, loop jejunostomy
- Laparostomy (ITU patient, multiple previous laparotomies, holes in bowel cannot be otherwise exteriorised).

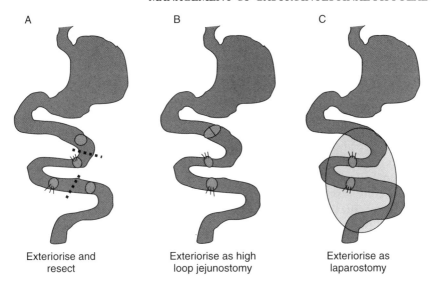

Figure 3.1 Surgical strategies to exteriorize the gut (see text for details).

The third manoeuvre is reserved for the very sick patient who has had two or three laparotomies, requires ventilation, renal and inotropic support. This technique of laparostomy, involves laying the abdomen open so that all of the defects of the gut are exteriorised to the surface (Figure 3.1C).[3] Laparostomy is essentially a first aid measure to try and arrest the septic illness. In these patients the question is not so much whether they will survive their laparostomies, but whether they will survive their multiple organ failure. In survivors, at the same time as the oxygen and inotropic support requirements decrease, the wound begins to cover with granulation tissue. Patients who worsen and die never seem to produce granulation tissue over the laparostomy. In improving patients the wound granulates and about six weeks later this sort of patient will no longer require organ support and the granulating wound will begin to contract. Such patients might still have quite extensive holes in the bowel that will ultimately need surgical closure but the context in which laparostomy is used is to try and get a live patient through the septic illness and create a situation where the abdomen can in time be re-accessed to close the fistulae.

Nutrition

Safe, complication-free nutrition is essential to maintain the patient whilst either awaiting spontaneous fistula closure or as the preliminary approach to surgical closure of the fistula. Enteral nutrition is to be preferred to parenteral nutrition if the majority of the gut is available for digestion and absorption of food. Intubation of the distal gut in an exposed non-healing fistula can be useful for establishing enteral nutrition if the distal gut is otherwise normal. In this author's experience the biggest rate-limiting step for successful enteral nutrition is abdominal pain and unfamiliarity of nursing staff with the treatment. An iso-osmolar food source is started and built up over two or three days. In this situation the nurses and the patient have to be confident that the abdominal pain will pass if enteral nutrition is persisted with.

Parenteral nutrition has been advocated as useful in the promotion of fistula closure by resting the injured bowel. There is no convincing evidence for this specific effect but clearly there is an absolute indication for parenteral nutrition if the fistula renders the majority of the gastrointestinal tract unavailable for enteric feeding. A typical parenteral feeding regimen should consist of 9 g nitrogen and 1400 kCal with suitable additives and electrolytes. Ideally, feed administration should be over a nocturnal 12-hour period allowing patient mobilisation during the day time. In practice the single greatest impediment to safe parenteral nutrition is line infection and sepsis.[4] Dedicated feeding lines managed by dedicated nursing staff are associated with the fewest line complications and the greatest line longevity.

Anatomy

The anatomy and location of both the fistula and the distal and proximal gastrointestinal tract should be established by a series of contrast studies. The distal studies are important in order to determine whether or not the gut might be suitable for enteral feeding and because the integrity of the distal gut is used to identify fistulae that are likely to close spontaneously. Fistulography through the external opening(s) is often able to demonstrate the origin of the fistula. Proximal and distal contrast studies are useful to demonstrate how much normal gut remains above and below the fistula and whether or not the distal obstruction beyond the fistula is present. The exact pattern of the contrast studies and their interpretation clearly requires close co-operation between clinicians and their radiologist colleagues.

Plan (or procedure)

Having eliminated sepsis, established complication-free nutrition and established fistula anatomy, including the anatomy of the distal GI tract, a plan of action to close the post-operative gastrointestinal fistula can be formulated. Conservative management of a post-operative fistula in the expectation of spontaneous closure can be pursued if the conditions outlined in Box 3.3 are met. It is probable that the vast majority of surgical fistulae close after two to six weeks of conservative management on the ward or in the ICU. Abscesses and obstruction prevent closure, and of course a fistula will not close if there is a drain or feeding tube through the fistula itself. Fistulae will also not close in the presence of primary Crohn's disease or cancer or if a fistula opening has healed to the skin.[2]

Box 3.3   Conditions required for conservative management

- No distal obstruction, no diseased gut
- No abscess, no foreign body (for example drain)
- No mucocutaneous continuity

The role of octreotide in early fistula closure in patients with post-operative enterocutaneous fistulae has been studied.[5] In the report by Scott *et al.*, 19 patients were randomised in a double blind fashion, to receive either 12 days of octreotide (100 µg tds) by subcutaneous injection, or 12 days of placebo injections. Fistula output for seven days before and during all 12 days of treatment was recorded. Fistula losses before entering the trial were similar for both the placebo group (n = 8) and those patients randomised to receive octreotide (n = 11) and there was no significant difference in fistula output during intervention. Fistula closure, defined as no fistula output for two successive days during the 12 day therapy period, was seen in only one patient given octreotide and in three patients who received placebo. This study showed that in patients with enterocutaneous fistulae, octreotide therapy was not associated with benefit.

If at the end of six weeks of conservative measures, spontaneous fistula closure does not occur, then it is likely that surgical reconstruction will be required to effect fistula closure.

Reconstruction

Surgical reconstruction of a post-operative gastrointestinal fistula is a challenging surgical exercise.[6] The key components of reconstruction include access to the peritoneal cavity, anastomosis of the GI tract and abdominal closure. Having got the patient relatively well, at what point should the decision be made to re-enter the abdomen to try and deal with the fistula itself? The timing for access to the abdomen in a patient with a post-operative fistula comes down to how long it takes to re-establish a new peritoneal cavity in the abdomen. This is usually around six to eight months after the last abdominal surgery. Clinically this is seen when a fistula originally embedded in granulation tissue starts demonstrating prolapse of the bowel.

The surgery often consists of several hours of picking away and undoing adhesions, finding and defining the intestinal anatomy, resecting the fistula and then carrying out an intestinal anastomosis. The next issue is to ensure the abdominal wall is closed over the anastomosis, since suture lines exposed on the abdomen simply break down again. In many patients, it is not too difficult to get abdominal closure, but the ones who have had laparostomies can often cause problems due to the size of the abdominal wall defect. The best approach is to achieve primary closure with double near and far prolene sutures and in the author's experience, using this technique there has been no need to ventilate any patients because of raised intra-abdominal pressure, re-fistulation has not been seen, and further surgery for an incisional hernia is also rarely seen.[7]

Rehabilitation

Post-operative fistulae are commonly managed conservatively with spontaneous resolution and patient discharge home being delayed by only a few weeks. In others post-operative fistulation can lead to weeks of life-threatening illness on an ICU with multiple organ failure, months in hospital with loss of enteric fluids into multiple bags, and repeated surgical intervention. In these latter circumstances disruption of physical, mental and social well being can be catastrophic for both the patient and their friends and family. Specialised nursing care and support is essential both for technical aspects of care – but also for coping and adjusting to the prolonged illness and body image consequences of post-operative fistulation. This support for patient and family is helped by patient support groups and may be required long after surgical reconstruction has been complete.

Outcome

The large majority of patients referred to the Intestinal Failure Unit at Hope Hospital are ultimately discharged home – only about 10% of those referred die after admission. The usual cause of death is multiple organ failure. Not surprisingly death is related to poor performance score, low serum albumin and age at referral. Older patients and patients with significant co-morbidity do particularly badly.

References

1   Williams N, Scott NA, Irving MH. Successful management of external duodenal fistula in a specialised unit. *Am J Surg* 1997;**173**(3):240–1.

2   Ayuk P, Williams N, Scott NA, Irving MH. The management of intra-abdominal abscesses in Crohn's disease. *Ann R Coll Surg Engl* 1996;**78**:5–10.

3   Carlson GL, Scott NA. Laparostomy and allied techniques. *Surgery* 1996; **14**(5):102–5.

4   Williams N, Scott NA, Irving MH. Catheter-related morbidity in patients on home parenteral nutrition: implications for small bowel transplantation. *Ann Roy Coll Surg Engl* 1994;**76**(6):384–6.

5   Scott NA, Finnegan S, Irving MH. Octreotide and post-operative enterocutaneous fistulae: a controlled prospective study. *Acta Gastroenterol Belg* 1993;**56**:266–70.

6   Scripcariu V, Carlson G, Bancewicz J, Irving MH, Scott NA. Reconstructive abdominal operations after laparostomy and multiple repeat laparotomies for severe intra-abdominal infection. *Br J Surg* 1994;**81**:1475–8.

7   A-Malik R, Scott NA. Double near and far prolene suture closure: a technique for abdominal wall closure after laparostomy. *Br J Surg* 2001;**88**:146–7.

4: The gut as the motor of organ failure

JOHN C MARSHALL

Introduction

Data from a large number of published human studies support the hypothesis that the gastrointestinal tract contributes to morbidity and mortality in critically ill patients on the intensive care unit (ICU). Changes in proximal gut flora in the critically ill patient predict nosocomial infection with the same organism, while therapeutic measures targeting the gut clearly reduce rates of nosocomial infection and may have an impact on mortality. Modulation of the systemic inflammatory response through gut-derived measures has been no more successful than modulation of that response through more conventional systemic forms of mediator-directed therapy. But although the gastrointestinal tract is an important factor in nosocomial ICU-acquired infection, to what extent does infection *per se* alter outcome in critical illness? The aim of this article is to provide a background to the evolution of the concept that in the critically ill patient the gut and its interactions with the liver play an important role in the clinical picture commonly seen in critically ill patients.

History

The idea that the gastrointestinal tract plays a role in the pathogenesis of disease dates back to ancient Egypt. In the 1950s and 1960s Jacob Fine demonstrated a critical role for a factor of gastrointestinal origin in the pathogenesis of traumatic shock.[1] He provided compelling evidence for what he termed an intestinal factor in the pathogenesis of haemorrhagic shock. This factor was identified as bacterial endotoxin. The stage was set for the rebirth of interest in the gut as an occult influence, driving the phenomenon of sepsis and multiple organ failure in critically ill patients. About 15 years ago, Jonathan Meakins and this author proposed that the gastrointestinal tract might be considered to be the "motor" of multiple organ failure – that is, the unseen force which somehow drove the systemic inflammatory response in critically ill patients.[2] This suggestion arose from the observation that patients in the ICU commonly develop recurrent episodes of relatively trivial infections with organisms not normally thought of as being particularly virulent, such as coagulase-negative Staphylococci, Enterococci and Candida, in association with a florid septic response. In many cases patients appeared to be clinically septic but a focus of infection could not be identified. Ileus, abdominal distension, and jaundice were common features of this clinical syndrome, reminiscent of the clinical scenario of an intra-abdominal abscess.

Nosocomial infection

The normal indigenous flora of the human gastrointestinal tract comprises a remarkably complex yet stable aggregation of more than 400 separate species, living in a symbiotic relationship with the human host. The stability of the flora is maintained by gastric acidity, gut motility, bile, products of immune cells in the gut epithelium, and competition between micro-organisms for nutrients and intestinal binding sites. The indigenous flora forms a key component of normal host defences against infection by exogenous pathogens. The gut also contains an enormous amount of endotoxin – roughly a gram of endotoxin is present in the normal gut, substantially more than is needed to trigger an inflammatory response, and yet, under normal circumstances we thrive perfectly well.

ICU-acquired infection in association with progressive organ system dysfunction is an important cause of morbidity and mortality in critical illness. Critical illness is associated with striking changes in patterns of microbial colonisation, which are particularly well-described in the oropharynx and upper gastrointestinal tract. Pathological colonisation occurs with the same species which predominate in nosocomial infections, and descriptive studies have suggested that such colonisation is a risk factor for infection. In order to determine the prevalence of ICU-acquired infections and the risk factors for these infections, identify the predominant infecting organisms, and evaluate the relationship between ICU-acquired infection and mortality, Vincent et al. undertook a one-day point-prevalence study in 1 417 ICUs in 17 countries in Western Europe – the EPIC study.[3] All adult patients occupying an ICU bed over a 24-hour period were included – a total of 10 038 patient case reports. It was found that 4 501 (44·8%) of patients were infected, and 2 064 (20·6%) had an infection acquired on ICU. Pneumonia (46·9%), lower respiratory tract infection (17·8%), urinary tract infection (17·6%) and bloodstream infection (12%) were the most frequently reported. The most common micro-organisms were *Enterobacteriaceae* (34·4%), *Staphylococcus aureus* (30·1%), *Pseudomonas aeruginosa* (28·7%), coagulase-negative Staphylococci (19·1%), and fungi (17·1%). The authors concluded that ICU-acquired

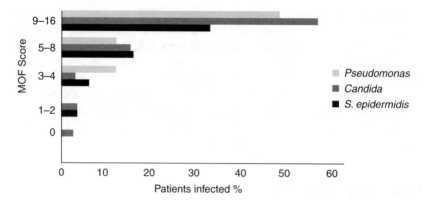

Figure 4.1 Association of organ failure and nosocomial infection with common pathogens encountered on the intensive care unit in 41 patients. See text for details. MOF = multiple organ failure score. Reproduced with permission by Harcourt International from Marshall JC, J Hosp Infect 1991;19:7–17.[4]

infection is common and often associated with microbiological isolates of resistant organisms.

A similar study in Canada revealed that nosocomial infection with common ICU pathogens was significantly associated with the severity of organ failure (Figure 4.1).[4] The association between proximal gastrointestinal colonisation and the development of nosocomial infection and multiple organ failure was investigated in a high risk population of critically ill surgical patients. Specimens of gastric and upper small bowel fluid were cultured and the severity of organ dysfunction was assessed using a numeric score in 41 surgical ICU patients. At least one episode of infection occurred in 33 patients and involved at least one organism concomitantly cultured from the upper gastrointestinal tract in all except three patients. The most common organisms causing infection were Candida, *Streptococcus faecalis, Pseudomonas*, and coagulase-negative Staphylococci and these were also the most common colonising species. ICU mortality was greater in patients colonised with *Pseudomonas*, and organ dysfunction was most marked in patients colonised with Candida, *Pseudomonas*, or *S. epidermidis*. These data suggest that the upper gastrointestinal tract is a reservoir of organisms which cause nosocomial infection. Pathological colonisation is also associated with the development of organ failure.

These studies were conducted at a time when prophylaxis with antacids was part of the routine management of ICU patients. It was observed that the pattern of colonisation of the gastrointestinal tract varied with the pH of the stomach.[5] Gram negative organisms only grew when the pH was above five. Below pH 5, *Pseudomonas* or other Gram negative organisms did not grow in the stomach, whereas at a pH >5 they did. In contrast, Gram positive organisms and fungi are relatively acid resistant, and continued to grow even at a pH as low as pH 1 (Figure 4.2).

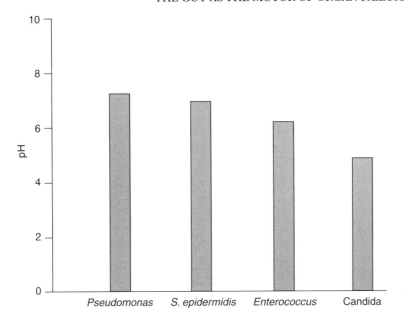

Figure 4.2 The relationship between gastric pH and colonisation with various organisms. See text for explanation. Reproduced with permission from Marshall JC, et al. Ann Surg *1993;218:111–19.*[5]

Bacterial translocation

Viable intact micro-organisms may enter the critically ill patient not only by aspiration of contaminated gastric or oropharyngeal secretions, but also across the gut mucosa and into mesenteric lymphatics, portal venous blood or the peritoneal cavity. This process of absorption of live organisms – from the gastrointestinal tract is termed bacterial translocation, and has been convincingly demonstrated in animal studies. Whether bacterial translocation occurs in humans has, until recently, been somewhat controversial. However, there are now enough data to establish that the gastrointestinal tract can serve as a portal of entry for micro-organisms through the process of bacterial translocation. Perhaps the most convincing data that micro-organisms can travel from the gut came from a study undertaken by several German surgeons in the late 1960s.[6] One of the surgeons drank 180 grams of a "liquid pulpy suspension" of live *Candida albicans* – about 10^{12} of the organisms whilst the other surgeon monitered the response. After two hours, it is reported, the subject felt very ill. *Candida* was isolated from his blood and urine. Other studies have shown that enteric bacteria can be isolated from ·tissues which are normally sterile. MacFie and colleagues[7] undertook a study of 279 surgical patients in whom cultures were obtained from the stomach, mesenteric lymph nodes, and sites of post-operative septic complications. Only 31% of patients had a sterile nasogastric aspirate; the most frequently identified organism was *Candida* spp. and the most common enteric organism cultured was *E. coli*. Multiple organisms were isolated in 39% of patients and occurred more frequently in patients aged over 70 years, those undergoing non-elective surgery, and those requiring proximal gastrointestinal surgery. Post-operative sepsis was also more common in these patients. Bacterial translocation occurred in 21% of patients but fungal translocation did not occur. It was concluded that proximal gut colonisation was associated with both increased bacterial translocation and septic morbidity.

To examine the spectrum of bacteria involved in translocation in surgical patients undergoing laparotomy and to determine the relation between nodal migration of bacteria and the development of post-operative septic complications O'Boyle *et al.* analysed mesenteric lymph nodes, serosal scrapings, and peripheral blood from 448 surgical patients undergoing laparotomy using standard microbiological techniques.[8] Bacterial translocation was identified in 69 patients (15·4%), the most common organism isolated being *Escherichia coli* (54%). Both enteric and non-enteric bacteria were isolated. Post-operative septic complications developed in 104 patients (23%) and enteric organisms were responsible in 74% of patients. In the patients who had evidence of bacterial translocation, 41% developed sepsis compared with only 14% in whom no organisms were cultured. This study again showed that bacterial translocation is associated with the development of post-operative sepsis in surgical patients. These data once more support the gut origin hypothesis of sepsis in humans.

Accumulating data suggest that a number of diseases are associated with microbial translocation in humans, including those in which the gut flora is altered, where there are changes in intestinal physiology, or which have been preceded by intestinal inflammation or ischaemia (Box 4.1).

The role of endotoxin

The translocation of viable micro-organisms into the body is one potential mechanism by which the gut might be fuelling the process of multiple organ failure and its associated manifestations of clinical sepsis and nosocomial infection. However, a number of studies have shown that in patients with life threatening infection, endotoxin can be isolated from blood – in patients with sepsis, meningococcaemia or peritonitis.[9–11] High rates of endotoxaemia are also seen in patients undergoing elective aortic aneurysm repair and patients undergoing cardiopulmonary bypass.[12,13] Niebauer and co-workers studied gut permeability and endotoxaemia in patients with oedema secondary to congestive heart failure.[14] Twenty patients with chronic heart failure with recent-onset peripheral oedema were compared with 20 stable non-oedematous patients with chronic heart failure and 14 healthy volunteers. Mean endotoxin concentrations were higher in patients with oedema than in stable patients and controls

---

Box 4.1 Diseases associated with microbial translocation

- Altered gut flora
    - Candida ingestion
    - Cirrhosis
    - Short bowel syndrome
    - Critical illness
- Altered intestinal physiology
    - Small bowel obstruction
    - Obstructive jaundice
- Intestinal inflammation
    - Inflammatory bowel disease
- Intestinal ischaemia
    - Aortic vascular disease
    - Cardiac arrest
    - Cardiopulmonary bypass
- Other
    - Trauma
    - Laparotomy
    - Home total parenteral nutrition
    - Small bowel transplantation

(Figure 4.3). Oedematous patients also had the highest concentrations of several cytokines. These findings suggest that endotoxin may trigger immune activation in patients with chronic heart failure during oedematous episodes. Since the only reservoir of significant quantities of endotoxin is the gastrointestinal tract, observations such as these suggest that the gut may also be an important site for the entry of endotoxin.

Cabie and colleagues[15] studied 14 patients undergoing abdominal aortic surgery to investigate whether endotoxaemia after mild ischaemia (bowel manipulation and aortic clamping) resulted in elevations in cytokine levels. Peri-operative endotoxin and cytokines were measured before clamping and after reperfusion, and compared in systemic and portal blood. Systemic levels of endotoxin and cytokines were also measured in a control group of seven patients undergoing internal carotid surgery. Endotoxin in portal blood was detectable in 36% of the patients undergoing aortic surgery after bowel manipulation, and in 71% after clamp release. Similar levels were observed in portal and systemic blood after clamp release. Circulating tumour necrosis factor α (TNFα) was observed in all patients

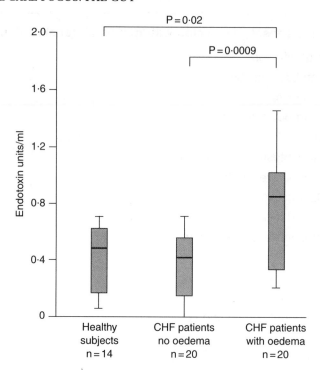

Figure 4.3 Serum concentrations of endotoxin in 14 healthy volunteers, 20 patients with chronic heart failure (CHF) without oedema and 20 patients with chronic heart failure plus oedema. Box and whisker plots show median, 25th and 75th percentile and range. Reproduced with permission from Elsevier Science (The Lancet *1999;353:1838–42*).[14]

undergoing aortic surgery. Levels of portal blood TNFα were higher than those in systemic blood after bowel manipulation as well as after reperfusion. These data suggest that there is generation of TNFα by the gut and gut epithelium which is absorbed into the portal venous system (Figure 4.4).

Another study investigated an alternate route for cytokine generation in patients with severe refractory multiple organ dysfunction.[16] Two men and two women were studied after 6–9 days of multiple organ dysfunction syndrome. The thoracic duct was cannulated, and samples of lymph and peripheral blood were obtained for assessment of lymph and serum levels of endotoxin, TNFα, interleukins-1β (IL-1β) and -6, and activation markers on T lymphocytes. Endotoxin and cytokine levels were low in lymph and serum, except for a mean lymph-to-serum ratio of 53·4 for IL-1β. There was phenotypical evidence of T-lymphocyte activation in both lymph and peripheral blood with increased lymph-to-peripheral blood ratios. These results provided evidence of the participation of gut-associated lymphatic tissue in the pathogenesis of the multiple organ dysfunction syndrome, suggesting that T-cell activation and cytokine production occur at the gut level.

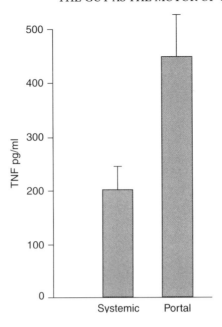

Figure 4.4 Tumour necrosis factor α (TNFα) concentrations in the portal venous and systemic circulation in seven patients undergoing aortic surgery. Reprinted from Cytokine, 5, Cabie et al., High levels of portal TNF-alpha during abdominal aortic surgery in man, 448–53, 1993 by permission of the publisher Academic Press.[15]

The gut immune system

Although this review has focused primarily on the gut and its role in the gastrointestinal system, the gut also contains the richest aggregate of immune tissue in the body (Box 4.2). A study conducted almost forty years ago used mice raised under germ-free conditions.[17] They had no indigenous gut flora; subsequent challenge with either *Staphylococcus aureus* or *Klebsiella* resulted in very high mortality, whereas conventional animals survived the

---

Box 4.2 Immune system of the gut

- Indigenous flora
- Gut epithelium
- Paneth cells
- M cells
- Gut associated lymphoid tissue
- Kupffer cells

---

challenge. Thus the presence of an intact gut flora provides immunity to challenge with common infecting pathogens. Interestingly germ-free mice were resistant to endotoxin, in contrast to conventional mice.

The more important role of the immune system of the gastrointestinal tract derives not from its ability to respond to challenge, but rather from its ability to not respond under circumstances that might evoke an immune response. Indeed the network of immune cells that line the gut exists in symbiosis with a potentially devastating indigenous microbial population, yet fails to respond. Epithelia of the intestinal tract characteristically maintain an inflammatory hyporesponsiveness toward the lumenal microflora. Transgenic mouse technology has revealed that animals with defined immune defects develop intestinal inflammation, presumably because they are no longer tolerant to their gut flora, and instead respond to that flora as though it were an antigen.

Neish and co-workers[18] reported the identification of non-virulent *Salmonella* strains whose direct interaction with model human epithelia attenuate the synthesis of inflammatory effector molecules elicited by diverse pro-inflammatory stimuli. This immunosuppressive effect involved inhibition of the inhibitory sub-unit of the transcription factor, nuclear factor kappa B (NFκB) by preventing ubiquitination of IκB, a process necessary for degradation of IκB and activation of NFκB, leading to the expression of many inflammatory mediators including cytokines and adhesion molecules. This study suggests that prokaryotic determinants could be responsible for the unique tolerance of the gastrointestinal mucosa to pro-inflammatory stimuli.

It has been suggested that a reduced microbial stimulation during infancy and early childhood might impair the development of tolerance in the immune system of the gut. To test the hypothesis that allergic disease among children may be associated with differences in their intestinal microflora in two countries with a low (Estonia) and a high (Sweden) prevalence of allergy, Bjorksten *et al.* undertook a study of 29 Estonian and 33 Swedish 2-year-old children.[19] Samples of faeces were serially diluted and grown under anaerobic conditions. The allergic children in Estonia and Sweden were less often colonised with lactobacilli as compared with the non-allergic. In contrast, the allergic children harboured higher counts of aerobic micro-organisms, particularly coliforms and *Staphylococcus aureus*. The proportions of aerobic bacteria of the intestinal flora were also higher in the allergic children, while the converse was true for anaerobes. Similarly, in the allergic children the proportions of coliforms were higher and bacteroides lower than in the non-allergic children. Thus differences in the indigenous intestinal flora might affect the development and priming of the immune system in early childhood, similar to what has been shown in animal studies. The role of intestinal microflora in relation to the development of infant immunity and the possible consequences for allergic diseases later in life requires further study, particularly since intervention by the administration of probiotic bacteria is possible.

Impairment of cell-mediated immunity is both a common manifestation of critical illness and a potential cause of increased infectious morbidity and mortality. The mechanisms responsible for alterations in systemic immune regulation are incompletely understood, although monocytes and macrophages appear to play a central role. It has been shown that infusion of Gram negative organisms into the portal vein, but not into the systemic circulation, induces suppression of delayed hypersensitivity responsiveness *in vivo* and of mitogen-stimulated lymphocyte proliferation *in vitro*.[20] Rats received killed *Pseudomonas aeruginosa* via the inferior vena cava or the portal vein and were killed 24 hours later, and the mitogen-driven proliferative responses of isolated splenocytes were assayed. Portal infusion resulted in significant suppression of mitogen-induced proliferative responses in comparison to systemically-infused animals, or to non-operated controls (Figure 4.5). Suppression was shown to be a consequence of the release of a soluble suppressive factor from splenic adherent cells. The stimulus for the release of this factor was not endotoxin, but a second factor released from the liver.

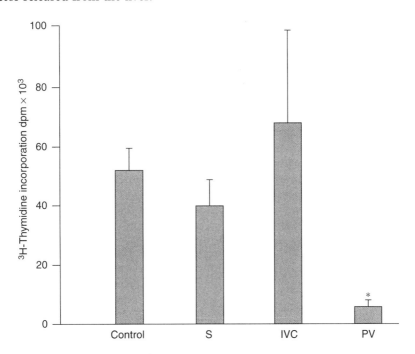

Figure 4.5 In vitro *incorporation of ^3H thymidine in Concanavalin A stimulated splenocytes from rats infused with killed* Pseudomonas aeruginosa *into either inferior vena cava (IVC) or the portal vein (PV) or systemically (S). Boxes are the mean of 10 replicate experiments. Reproduced with permission from Marshall JC, et al. J Surg Res 1993;55:14–20.*[20]

Intestinal decontamination with streptomycin sulphate and bacitracin followed by oral feeding with a streptomycin-resistant strain of *Escherichia coli* produces single organism colonisation of the gastrointestinal tract. Using this rat model, the rate of bacterial translocation at day three increased from 6% to 90%. Cell-associated pro-coagulant activity was measured in the mononuclear cell population of mesenteric lymph nodes, in portal and systemic blood, and in hepatic non-parenchymal cells.[21] The pro-coagulant activity of mesenteric lymph node mononuclear cells was significantly greater in colonised than in control animals at day three but not at days one or six. Pro-coagulant activity of hepatic non-parenchymal cells was elevated in colonised animals at days three and six compared with control animals. These studies provided evidence that bacterial translocation can induce cell activation at sites remote from the gastrointestinal tract and may therefore contribute to the pathogenesis of multiple organ failure.

The interaction of the gut flora and the gut immune system serves not so much to protect against bacteria in the gut, but to limit innate immunity to those bacteria that are present. In critically ill patients if either the gut flora or the gut immune system is altered, systemic inflammation may be induced.

Feeding and nosocomial infection

If the gut is the motor of multiple organ failure, then what is the fuel? Enteral nutrients maintain normal immune status in the gut and intestinal tract, and the incidence of pneumonia, intra-abdominal abscesses, and line infections can all be reduced in trauma victims by feeding.[22] More recently the concept has been applied to patients with acute necrotising pancreatitis: four studies randomising patients to parenteral nutrition versus enteral nutrition show that patients who are fed enterally have lower mortality than those patients who are fed parenterally.[23-26] One of the easiest ways to blunt the inflammatory response and improve outcome is to feed the gut.

Decontaminating the gut

Animal data from mice given oral antibiotics with anti-anaerobic activity show a striking increase in the number of bacteria that can be isolated from the caecum. In a study by Berg, there were one hundred thousand times as many *E. coli* in the caecum of mice treated with clindamycin than in untreated animals.[27] In those animals which received the antibiotic, 100% had demonstrable bacterial translocation to mesenteric lymph nodes.

There is also convincing evidence in humans for the use of selective digestive tract decontamination (SDD). The SDD combination (Box 4.3) targets only aerobic Gram negative organisms and fungi, leaving the anaerobes and Gram positive bacteria intact. To determine the comparative efficacy of selective decontamination of the digestive tract in critically ill

---

Box 4.3 Selective decontamination of the digestive tract

- TOPICAL

Polymyxin B	Targets aerobic Gram negatives
Tobramycin	Targets aerobic Gram negatives
Amphotericin B	Targets fungi

- SYSTEMIC

Cefotaxime	Targets community-acquired Gram positives and Gram negatives; given for 3 to 4 days

Topical agents are administered as a suspension via the nasogastric tube, and as a paste to the oropharynx

---

surgical and medical patients, and in selected subgroups of surgical patients with pancreatitis, major burn injury, and those undergoing major elective surgery and transplantation, Nathens and Marshall undertook a meta-analysis evaluating the efficacy of selective decontamination of the digestive tract in human subjects.[28] Mortality was significantly reduced with the use of selective decontamination of the digestive tract in critically ill surgical patients, whereas no such effect was seen in critically ill medical patients. Rates of pneumonia were reduced in both medical and surgical patients, but bacteraemia was reduced only in surgical patients.

Summary

The microbial flora of the normal gut is complex, yet remarkably constant over time. The relative sterility of the upper gut is maintained by multiple factors including gastric acid, bile salts, normal motility and mucosal IgA, while the lower gut is densely colonised with a complex flora. An intact Gram negative flora is a prerequisite for normal immunological maturation. On the other hand, overgrowth of the gut, particularly by Gram negative bacteria or fungi, facilitates the translocation of bacteria into the host, and results in suppression of T-cell responses and altered hepatic Kupffer cell function. Bacterial overgrowth and the consequences of the interactions of this potentially pathogenic flora with the gut immune system may contribute to the septic state in critical illness, and to the syndrome of multiple organ failure. Prevention of pathological gut colonisation reduces the rate of nosocomial infection in critically ill patients, and even reduces mortality risk. Conventional approaches to infectious diseases have focused on eradicating micro-organisms, but studies in critically ill patients suggest that the relationship between bacteria and the host is better understood as a symbiotic one and that preservation, rather than elimination, of the indigenous flora provides the greatest promise of clinical benefit in a highly vulnerable patient population.

References

1 Fine J, Frank ED, Ravin HA, Rutenberg SH, Schweinburg FB. The bacterial factor in traumatic shock. *N Engl J Med* 1959;**260**:214–20.
2 Carrico CJ, Meakins JL, Marshall JC, Fry D, Maier RV. Multiple organ failure syndrome. The gastrointestinal tract: the motor of MOF. *Arch Surg* 1986;**121**:196–208.
3 Vincent JL, Bihari DJ, Suter PM, *et al.* The prevalence of nosocomial infection in intensive care units in Europe. Results of the European Prevalence of Infection in Intensive Care (EPIC) Study. EPIC International Advisory Committee. *J Am Med Assoc* 1995;**274**:639–44.
4 Marshall JC. The ecology and immunology of the gastrointestinal tract in health and critical illness. *J Hosp Infect* 1991;**19**:7–17.
5 Marshall JC, Christou NV, Meakins JL. The gastrointestinal tract. The "undrained abscess" of multiple organ failure. *Ann Surg* 1993;**218**:111–19.
6 Krause W, Matheis H, Wulf K. Fungaemia and funguria after oral administration of *Candida albicans*. *Lancet* 1969;**1**:598–9.
7 MacFie J, O'Boyle C, Mitchell CJ, Buckley PM, Johnstone D, Sudworth P. Gut origin of sepsis: a prospective study investigating associations between bacterial translocation, gastric microflora, and septic morbidity. *Gut* 1999;**45**:223–8.
8 O'Boyle CJ, MacFie J, Mitchell CJ, Johnstone D, Sagar PM, Sedman PC. Microbiology of bacterial translocation in humans. *Gut* 1998;**42**:29–35.
9 Opal SM, Scannon PJ, Vincent JL, *et al.* Relationship between plasma levels of lipopolysaccharide (LPS) and LPS-binding protein in patients with severe sepsis and septic shock. *J Infect Dis* 1999;**180**:1584–9.
10 Waage A, Brandtzaeg P, Halstensen A, Kierulf P, Espevik T. The complex pattern of cytokines in serum from patients with meningococcal septic shock. Association between interleukin 6, interleukin 1, and fatal outcome. *J Exp Med* 1989;**169**:333–8.
11 Hamilton G, Hofbauer S, Hamilton B. Endotoxin, TNF-alpha, interleukin-6 and parameters of the cellular immune system in patients with intraabdominal sepsis. *Scand J Infect Dis* 1992;**24**:361–8.
12 Soong CV, Blair PH, Halliday MI, *et al.* Endotoxaemia, the generation of the cytokines and their relationship to intramucosal acidosis of the sigmoid colon in elective abdominal aortic aneurysm repair. *Eur J Vasc Surg* 1993;**7**:534–9.
13 Jansen PG, Te Velthuis H, Oudemans-Van Straaten HM, *et al.* Perfusion-related factors of endotoxin release during cardiopulmonary bypass. *Eur J Cardiothorac Surg* 1994;**8**:125–9.
14 Niebauer J, Volk HD, Kemp M, *et al.* Endotoxin and immune activation in chronic heart failure: a prospective cohort study. *Lancet* 1999;**353**:1838–42.
15 Cabie A, Farkas JC, Fitting C, *et al.* High levels of portal TNF-alpha during abdominal aortic surgery in man. *Cytokine* 1993;**5**:448–53.
16 Sanchez-Garcia M, Prieto A, Tejedor A, *et al.* Characteristics of thoracic duct lymph in multiple organ dysfunction syndrome. *Arch Surg* 1997;**132**:13–18.
17 Dubos RJ, Schaedler RW. The effect of the intestinal flora on the growth rate of mice, and their susceptibility to experimental infections. *J Exp Med* 1960;**111**:407–17.

18 Neish AS, Gewirtz AT, Zeng H, *et al*. Prokaryotic regulation of epithelial responses by inhibition of IkappaB-alpha ubiquitination. *Science* 2000;**289**: 1560–3.

19 Bjorksten B, Naaber P, Sepp E, Mikelsaar M. The intestinal microflora in allergic Estonian and Swedish 2-year-old children. *Clin Exp Allergy* 1999; **29**:342–6.

20 Marshall JC, Ribeiro MB, Chu PT, Rotstein OD, Sheiner PA. Portal endotoxemia stimulates the release of an immunosuppressive factor from alveolar and splenic macrophages. *J Surg Res* 1993;**55**:14–20.

21 Sullivan BJ, Swallow CJ, Girotti MJ, Rotstein OD. Bacterial translocation induces procoagulant activity in tissue macrophages. A potential mechanism for end-organ dysfunction. *Arch Surg* 1991;**126**:586–90.

22 Kudsk KA, Croce MA, Fabian TC, *et al*. Enteral versus parenteral feeding. Effects on septic morbidity after blunt and penetrating abdominal trauma. *Ann Surg* 1992;**215**:503–11.

23 McClave SA, Snider H, Owens N, Sexton LK. Clinical nutrition in pancreatitis. *Dig Dis Sci* 1997;**42**:2035–44.

24 Kalfarentzos F, Kehagias J, Mead N, Kokkinis K, Gogos CA. Enteral nutrition is superior to parenteral nutrition in severe acute pancreatitis: results of a randomized prospective trial. *Br J Surg* 1997;**84**:1665–9.

25 Windsor AC, Kanwar S, Li AG, *et al*. Compared with parenteral nutrition, enteral feeding attenuates the acute phase response and improves disease severity in acute pancreatitis. *Gut* 1998;**42**:431–5.

26 Pupelis G, Austrums E, Jansone A, Sprucs R, Wehbi H. Randomised trial of safety and efficacy of postoperative enteral feeding in patients with severe pancreatitis: preliminary report. *Eur J Surg* 2000;**166**:383–7.

27 Berg RD. Promotion of the translocation of enteric bacteria from the gastrointestinal tracts of mice by oral treatment with penicillin, clindamycin, or metronidazole. *Infect Immun* 1981;**33**:854–61.

28 Nathens AB, Marshall JC. Selective decontamination of the digestive tract in surgical patients: a systematic review of the evidence. *Arch Surg* 1999;**134**: 170–6.

5: Mesenteric ischaemia

ULF HAGLUND, HELEN F GALLEY

Introduction

In this article the physiology of the intestinal circulation of importance for the understanding of intestinal ischaemia is briefly outlined. The key to our understanding and successful treatment of intestinal ischaemia lies in a better knowledge of this physiology. The potential for intestinal vasoconstriction causing non-occlusive intestinal ischaemia is discussed, as is the role of the reperfusion component of ischaemic injury. Maintenance of the mucosal cell barrier is essential in preventing the translocation of bacteria and endotoxin into the portal circulation and mesenteric lymphatics and the importance of this in the critically ill is addressed.

Causes of ischaemia

Depending on the severity and duration, intestinal ischaemia induces injury ranging from minor changes in permeability in mucosal capillaries to severe infarction. Two events cause intestinal injury during ischaemia – hypoxia during the ischaemia itself and generation of free radicals upon reperfusion. Intestinal ischaemia occurs when the metabolic demand of the tissue supersedes the delivery of oxygen as a result of inadequate systemic blood flow or local vascular abnormalities. The small intestine is capable of autoregulation of blood flow over a wide range of perfusion pressures. In addition, despite reduced flow, intestinal oxygen uptake is maintained by increases in oxygen extraction provided blood flow remains above a critical level. Oxygen uptake only becomes flow limited when blood flow falls below this level. The consequence of this protective compensatory mechanism, is such that even relatively prolonged reductions in blood flow do not cause even mild injury. Thus moderately mild reductions in intestinal perfusion pressure and/or blood flow cause little evidence of injury.

Ischaemic bowel disease occurs more often in the elderly since in older patients the vascular supply can frequently be compromised. The clinical manifestations are varied, depending on the site of vascular occlusion and the extent of the resulting bowel necrosis.

Mesenteric vasculature

The blood flow to the splanchnic organs is derived from three main arterial trunks, the coeliac artery, the superior mesenteric artery and the inferior mesenteric artery. The coeliac artery supplies blood to the stomach and duodenum, the superior mesenteric artery supplies blood to the gut from the duodenum to the transverse colon, and the inferior mesenteric artery is responsible for blood supply to the colon from the transverse colon to the rectum. Each of these three arterial trunks supplies blood flow to its specific section of the gastrointestinal tract through a vast network (Figure 5.1).

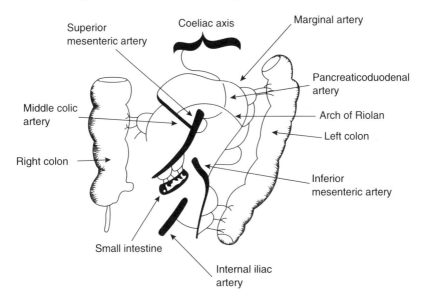

Figure 5.1 Schematic representation of the splanchnic circulation.

Since blood can reach a specific segment of gut via more than one route, this provides an effective protection against ischaemia, and additional vascular protection is obtained from connections between the three arterial systems. Communication between the coeliac system and the superior mesenteric system generally occurs via the superior pancreaticoduodenal and the inferior pancreaticoduodenal arteries. The superior mesenteric and inferior mesenteric systems are joined by the arch of Riolan and the marginal artery of Drummond, vessels that connect the middle colic artery (a branch of the superior mesenteric artery) and the left colic artery (a branch of the inferior mesenteric artery). In addition, communication also exists between the inferior mesenteric artery and branches of the internal iliac arteries via the rectum.

In chronic vascular insufficiency, blood flow to an individual system can be maintained through these collateral connections even when an arterial trunk is completely obstructed and the calibre of these connections can vary considerably. It is not uncommon to find that one or even two arterial trunks are completely occluded without any symptoms in patients with chronic vascular disease. There are even reports of occlusion of all three arterial trunks in patients who are still able to maintain their splanchnic circulation. However, in up to 30% of people, the collateral connections between the superior and inferior mesenteric arteries, via the arch of Riolan and the marginal artery of Drummond, can be weak or non existent, making the area of the splenic flexure particularly vulnerable to acute ischaemia.

Splanchnic blood flow

The mesenteric circulation receives approximately 30% of the cardiac output. Mesenteric blood flow is less in the fasting state and is increased with feeding. Blood flow through the coeliac and superior mesenteric trunks is about equal (approximately 700 ml/min in the adult) and is twice the blood flow through the inferior mesenteric trunk. Blood flow distribution within the gut wall is not uniform, and it varies between the mucosa and the muscularis. The mucosa has the highest metabolic rate and receives about 70% of the mesenteric blood flow. The small bowel receives the most blood, followed by the colon and then the stomach.

Many factors are involved in the control of gastrointestinal blood flow. Vascular resistance is proportional to the fourth power of the radius of the vessel such that the smaller the artery, the greater its ability to effect vascular resistance. It is known that the majority of blood flow control occurs at the level of the arterioles, the so-called resistance vessels. Very little control of blood flow occurs at the level of the large arterial trunks. In fact, the diameter of these large arterial trunks can be compromised by 75% before blood flow is reduced. Additional control of blood flow occurs at the level of the pre-capillary sphincter. In the fasting state only one-fifth of capillary beds are open, leaving a tremendous reserve to meet any increased metabolic demands.

Among the most important control mechanisms of splanchnic blood flow are the sympathetic nervous system, humoral factors and local factors. The sympathetic nervous system through α adrenergic receptors plays a role in maintaining the basal vascular tone and in mediating vasoconstriction. Beta-adrenergic activity appears to mediate vasodilation, and it appears that the antrum of the stomach may be particularly rich in these β receptors. Humoral factors involved in the regulation of gastrointestinal blood flow include catecholamines, and perhaps more important the renin-angiotensin system and vasopressin. These latter humoral systems may play a particularly important role in shock states. Local factors appear to be mainly involved in the matching of tissue blood flow to the metabolic demand. An increased metabolic rate may produce a decreased pO_2, increased pCO_2 and an increased level of adenosine, each of which can mediate a hyperaemic response.

The vascular endothelium is a source for potent vasoactive substances, such as the vasodilator nitric oxide and the vasoconstrictor endothelin. Burgener and co-workers[1] recently showed that endothelin-1 blockade in a pig acute cardiac failure model improved mesenteric but not renal perfusion, illustrating the regional importance of endothelin-1-induced vasoconstriction. Importantly, endothelin-1 blockade restored mucosal blood flow and oxygenation, which might be particularly interesting considering the implications for maintenance of mucosal barrier integrity in low output states.

Classification of intestinal ischaemia

Many clinicians broadly classify intestinal ischaemia into acute or chronic disease. However, classification of ischaemic bowel disease is not always applicable because certain acute events can become a chronic condition. Since the extent of intestinal ischaemia and the pathological consequences depend on the size and the location of the occluded or hypoperfused intestinal blood vessel or vessels, it is perhaps more useful to classify ischaemic bowel disease according to whether vessels are hypoperfused or occluded. Accordingly, intestinal ischaemia may result from occlusion or hypoperfusion of a large mesenteric vessel (for example the mesenteric artery or vein) or from occlusion or hypoperfusion of smaller intramural intestinal vessels. In each of these situations the intestinal ischaemia can be acute or chronic. In addition, vessel occlusion or hypoperfusion can be the result of a mechanical intraluminal obstruction such as an embolus or thrombus or can be non-occlusive ischaemia as the result of decreased blood flow due to vasospasm, increased blood viscosity or hypotension. A clinically important further classification is whether the ischaemia-induced necrosis is transmural (gangrenous ischaemia) leading to peritonitis, or remains intramural (non-gangrenous ischaemia) resulting in localised disease.

Pathophysiology of intestinal ischaemia

Intestinal ischaemia occurs when the metabolic demand of the tissue exceeds oxygen delivery. Obviously, many factors can be involved in this mismatch of oxygen need and demand. These include:

- the general haemodynamic state
- the degree of atherosclerosis

- extent of collateral circulation
- neurogenic, humoral, or local control mechanisms of vascular resistance
- abnormal products of cellular metabolism before and after reperfusion of an ischaemic segment.

Acute occlusion or hypoperfusion of a large mesenteric vessel usually results in transmural (gangrenous) ischaemia of the small bowel and/or colon. On the other hand, acute occlusion of the smaller intramural vessel usually results in intramural (non-gangrenous) ischaemia. However, there are exceptions in both cases, depending on the severity of occlusion or hypoperfusion.

As previously mentioned, the mucosa is the most metabolically active tissue layer of the gut wall and is the first tissue layer to be affected by ischaemia. The earliest event in intestinal ischaemia is changes at the tip of the intestinal villi. With ongoing total ischaemia ultrastructural changes begin within 10 minutes and cellular damage is extensive by 30 minutes. Sloughing of the villi tips in the small bowel and the superficial mucosal layer of the colon is followed by oedema, sub-mucosal haemorrhage and eventual transmural necrosis. The intestinal response to ischaemia is first characterised by a hypermotility state causing severe pain, even though the ischaemic damage may still be limited to the mucosa at this stage. As the ischaemia progresses, motor activity will cease and gut mucosal permeability will increase, leading to an increase in bacterial translocation. With transmural extension of the ischaemia, the patient will develop visceral and parietal inflammation resulting in peritonitis.

Vasospasm

An important factor often responsible for, or aggravating, intestinal ischaemia is the phenomenon of vasospasm. It has shown that both occlusive and non-occlusive forms of arterial ischaemia can result in prolonged vasospasm, even after the occlusion has been removed or the perfusion pressure restored. Such vasospasm may persist for several hours, resulting in prolonged ischaemia. The mechanism responsible for this vasospasm is not clearly defined, but there is some evidence that the potent vasoconstrictor endothelin may be involved.[2]

Reperfusion injury

A second factor that may be responsible for accentuating ischaemic damage is reperfusion injury. As mentioned above, there are two components generally thought to contribute to the mucosal injury associated with intestinal ischaemia – these are hypoxia during the ischaemic period, and oxygen-derived free radicals generated during reperfusion. The hypoxia of

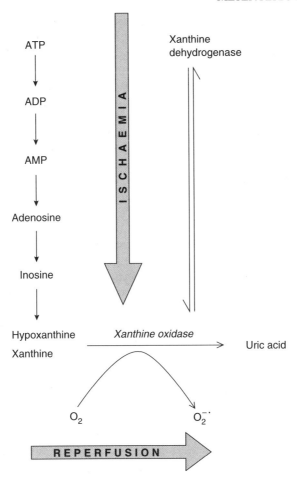

Figure 5.2 Activation of xanthine oxidase during ischaemia and the formation of superoxide anion upon reperfusion.

the intestinal villi during the ischaemic period is exaggerated by the countercurrent mechanism.[3] The oxygen-derived free radical hypothesis predicts that the mucosal injury results from reperfusion of ischaemic tissue through production of superoxide from xanthine oxidase (Figure 5.2).[4–6] The generation of oxygen-derived free radicals at reperfusion has been well demonstrated in the laboratory, where following moderate intestinal ischaemia, it has been shown to be responsible for a greater degree of cellular damage than that brought about during the actual ischaemic period. Parks and Granger undertook a systematic histological evaluation of the time course of development of mucosal lesions during moderate intestinal ischaemia and following reperfusion in a regional ischaemia model.[4] Reperfusion after three hours of regional hypotension reduced mean mucosal thickness from $1022\,\mu m$ to $504\,\mu m$, due mostly to a reduction in villus height. The change in mucosal thickness was much smaller when the bowel was subjected to three hours of ischaemia without reperfusion. In addition, the mucosal injury produced by three hours' ischaemia and one hour of reperfusion was more severe than that produced by four hours' ischaemia without reperfusion. The results of this study suggest that most of the tissue damage produced by the widely employed regional hypotension model, where intestinal blood flow is decreased to 25–30% of control, occurs due to reperfusion rather than ischaemia. Subsequent work showed a protective effect of xanthine oxidase inhibition, confirming the role of xanthine oxidase activation.[5]

It is not known what role ischaemia-reperfusion injury plays in humans with occlusive or non-occlusive disease. In a rat model, experimental gut ischaemia and reperfusion was followed by acute lung and liver injury[7,8] and was associated with xanthine oxidase activation.[8] Xanthine oxidase activation has also been demonstrated in patients with sepsis.[9] In total or near total intestinal ischaemia the reperfusion component of the tissue injury is much less if not non-existent.[3,5] However, tissue injury at reperfusion has been reported after partial ischaemia and total intestinal ischaemia may be followed by reperfusion injury if there is no concomitant congestion and if ischaemic injury is not too extensive.[10]

Ischaemia and sepsis

The mesenteric haemodynamic response to shock is characteristic and profound; this vasoconstrictive response disproportionately affects both the mesenteric organs and the organism as a whole. Vasoconstriction of post-capillary mesenteric venules and veins, mediated largely by the α adrenergic receptors of the sympathetic nervous system, can effect an "autotransfusion" of up to 30% of the total circulating blood volume, supporting cardiac filling pressures, and thereby sustaining cardiac output at virtually no cost in nutrient flow to the mesenteric organs. Under conditions of decreased cardiac output, selective vasoconstriction of the afferent mesenteric arterioles serves to sustain total systemic vascular resistance, thereby maintaining systemic arterial pressure and sustaining the perfusion of non-mesenteric organs at the expense of mesenteric organ perfusion. This markedly disproportionate response of the mesenteric resistance vessels is largely independent of the sympathetic nervous system and variably related to vasopressin, but mediated primarily by the renin-angiotensin axis. The extreme of this response can lead to gastric stress erosions, non-occlusive mesenteric ischaemia, ischaemic -colitis, -hepatitis, -cholecystitis, and/or -pancreatitis. Septic shock can produce decreased or increased mesenteric perfusion, but is characterised by increased oxygen consumption exceeding the capacity of mesenteric oxygen delivery, resulting in ischaemia and consequent tissue injury. Mesenteric organ injury from ischaemia/reperfusion due to any form of shock can lead to a triggering of systemic inflammatory response syndrome, and ultimately to multiple organ dysfunction syndrome. The mesenteric vasculature is therefore a major target and a primary determinant of the systemic response to shock.

Bacterial translocation

The concept of translocation of bacteria or their products from the lumen of the intestine into the mesenteric circulation and mesenteric lymph nodes was established several years ago.[11] Studies on the biology of endotoxin proposed a relationship between increases in intestinal permeability associated with translocation of endotoxin and Gram negative bacteria and the potential for remote organ failure following haemorrhagic shock, chemical injury, trauma and burns. Unfortunately, initial clinical work was contradictory. Rush *et al.* related endotoxaemia and bacteraemia to later organ failure and mortality in severely injured patients.[12] However a subsequent study failed to demonstrate bacteria or endotoxin in the portal blood of severely injured patients.[13]

The role of cytokines

Recent studies have increased the understanding of gut barrier failure and the pathophysiology of sepsis and multiple organ dysfunction beyond original bacterial translocation and xanthine oxidase activation. Shock, trauma, or sepsis-induced gut injury can result in the generation of cytokines and other pro-inflammatory mediators in the gut[14] and the mesenteric lymph may be the route of delivery of inflammatory mediators from the gut to remote organs.[15] Toxic products were demonstrated in mesenteric lymph but not in the systemic or portal circulation.[15] Deitch *et al.* showed that lung injury after haemorrhagic shock and increased endothelial cell permeability appears to be caused by toxic factors carried in the mesenteric lymph.[16] Another study showed that gut-derived lymph promotes haemorrhagic shock-induced lung injury through up-regulation of the adhesion molecule P-selectin.[17] Division or ligation of lymphatics in the gut mesentery before induction of shock prevented this increase in lung permeability and limited shock-induced pulmonary neutrophil recruitment.[14,16,17]

Thus gut-derived lymph has a significant role in the generation of remote organ injury after shock, particularly lung injury. Factors produced in the gut are transported to the systemic circulation by mesenteric lymphatics emptying into the thoracic duct, which subsequently drains into the systemic and particularly pulmonary circulation. Gut ischaemia reflected by gastric tonometry is a better predictor of the development of acute lung injury than global indexes of oxygen delivery or consumption in critically ill patients.[18]

Therapeutic approaches in the critically ill

Therapeutic approaches to treat or prevent gut ischaemia and reperfusion injury in critically ill patients remain a matter for debate. Sims and colleagues[19] recently reported that intravenous Ringer's ethyl pyruvate was more effective than pyruvate in ameliorating mucosal permeability changes after reperfusion injury in a rat model (Figure 5.3). Other approaches have included hypothermia, prostaglandin E, and modulation of blood flow by diltiazem, nitric oxide donors, or angiotensin-converting enzyme inhibition.[20] In addition, interference with neutrophil function or adhesion decreased the degree of ischaemia/reperfusion mucosal injury in a rat model.[21]

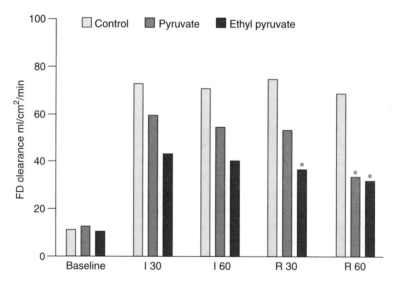

*Figure 5.3 Effect of treatment with Ringer's pyruvate or Ringer's ethyl pyruvate solution on intestinal mucosal permeability to 4000 Da fluorescein isothiocyanate dextran in rats subjected to mesenteric ischaemia and reperfusion. Control animals received lactated Ringer's solution. The time points are baseline (before the onset of ischaemia), I 30 and I 60 (after 30 and 60 mins of ischaemia), and R 30 and R 60 (after 30 and 60 min of reperfusion). *p < 0·05 compared with the time-matched value in the control group. Reproduced with permission from Sims CA, et al. Crit Care Med 2001;29:1513–18.[19]*

Xia and colleagues[22] showed that the antioxidant enzyme superoxide dismutase increased cellular energy stores and decreased mucosal injury after reperfusion and, as mentioned above, inhibition of xanthine oxidase has also been shown to attenuate mucosal cell injury in an animal model.[6]

Intraluminal treatments have the advantage of being able to deliver active agent directly to the mucosal cells and this may be delivered at concentrations higher than that tolerated in the circulation with fewer systemic side effects. Intraluminal therapy with sodium pyruvate, a 3-carbon compound known to inhibit superoxide production, attenuates reperfusion mucosal injury in the rat.[23] Intraluminal administration of L-arginine or a nitric oxide donor in rats prior to mesenteric artery occlusion decreased mucosal permeability and improved survival, presumably by increasing nitric oxide-mediated blood flow.[24]

Conclusion

Mucosal injury develops rapidly in the gut after shock or splanchnic ischaemia due to decreased mucosal blood flow, increased short-circuiting of oxygen in the mucosal countercurrent exchanger, and increased oxygen demand. In addition, reperfusion injury may also contribute as a result of increased generation of oxygen-derived radicals via xanthine oxidase activation. As a consequence of increased permeability of the intestinal mucosal barrier, translocation of bacteria and bacterial endotoxin also takes place.

A significant limitation of many studies investigating therapeutic approaches is the use of pre-treatment, i.e. before the onset of the ischaemia and reperfusion injury. In the critically ill the earliest opportunity for medical intervention may be hours after the onset of gut ischaemia. The ideal approach to ischaemia/reperfusion injury is prevention through injury avoidance and rapid resuscitation but randomised controlled trials are essential. Combinations of intravenous and intraluminal agents are perhaps the best approach.

References

1   Burgener D, Laesser M, Treggiari-Venzi M, *et al.* Endothelin-1 blockade corrects mesenteric hypoperfusion in a porcine low cardiac output model. *Crit Care Med* 2001;**29**:1615–20.

2   Murch SH, Braegger CP, Sessa WC, MacDonald TT. High endothelin-1 immunoreactivity in Crohn's disease and ulcerative colitis. *Lancet* 1992;**339**: 381–5.

3   Granger DN, Hollwarth ME, Parks DA. Ischemia-reperfusion injury: role of oxygen-derived free radicals. *Acta Physiol Scand Suppl* 1986;**548**:47–63.

4   Parks DA, Granger DN. Contributions of ischemia and reperfusion to mucosal lesion formation. *Am J Physiol* 1986;**250**:G749–53.

5   Haglund U, Bulkley GB, Granger DN. On the pathophysiology of intestinal ischaemic injury. *Acta Chir Scand* 1987;**153**:321–4.

6   Granger DN, McCord JM, Parks DA, Hollwarth ME. Xanthine oxidase inhibitors attenuate ischemia-induced vascular permeability changes in the cat intestine. *Gastroenterology* 1986;**90**:80–4.

7   Schmeling DJ, Caty MG, Oldham KT, Guice KS, Hinshaw DB. Evidence for neutrophil-related acute lung injury after intestinal ischemia-reperfusion. *Surgery* 1989;**106**:195–201.
8   Poggetti RS, Moore FA, Moore EE, Koeike K, Banerjee A. Simultaneous liver and lung injury following gut ischemia is mediated by xanthine oxidase. *J Trauma* 1992;**32**:723–7.
9   Galley HF, Davies MJ, Webster NR. Xanthine oxidase activity and free radical generation in patients with sepsis syndrome. *Crit Care Med* 1996;**24**:1649–53.
10 Park PO, Haglund U, Bulkley GB, Fält K. The sequence of development of tissue injury after strangulation ischemia and reperfusion. *Surgery* 1990;**107**: 575–80.
11 Deitch EA, Berg R. Bacterial translocation from the gut: a mechanism of infection. *J Burn Care Rehabil* 1987;**8**(6):475–82.
12 Rush BF Jr, Sori AJ, Murphy TF, Smith S, Machiedo GW. Endotoxemia and bacteremia during hemorrhagic shock: The link between trauma and sepsis? *Ann Surg* 1988;**207**:549–54.
13 Moore FA, Moore EE, Poggetti R, *et al*. Gut bacterial translocation via the portal vein: A clinical perspective with major torso trauma. *J Trauma* 1991;**31**:629–38.
14 Sambol JT, Xu DZ, Adams CA, Magnotti LJ, Deitch EA. Mesenteric lymph duct ligation provides long term protection against hemorrhagic shock-induced lung injury. *Shock* 2000;**14**:416–20.
15 Magnotti LJ, Upperman JS, Xu DZ, Lu Q, Deitch EA. Gut-derived mesenteric lymph but not portal blood increases endothelial cell permeability and promotes lung injury after hemorrhagic shock. *Ann Surg* 1998;**228**:518–27.
16 Deitch EA, Adams C, Lu Q, Xu DZ. A time course study of the protective effect of mesenteric lymph duct ligation on hemorrhagic shock-induced pulmonary injury and the toxic effects of lymph from shocked rats on endothelial cell monolayer permeability. *Surgery* 2001;**129**:39–47.
17 Adams CA Jr, Sambol JT, Xu DZ, Lu Q, Granger DN, Deitch EA. Hemorrhagic shock induced up-regulation of P-selectin expression is mediated by factors in mesenteric lymph and blunted by mesenteric lymph duct interruption. *J Trauma* 2001;**51**:625–31.
18 Ivatury RR, Simon RJ, Islam S, Fueg A, Rohman M, Stahl WM. A prospective randomized study of end points of resuscitation after major trauma: Global oxygen transport indices versus organ specific gastric mucosal pH. *J Am Coll Surg* 1996;**183**:145–54.
19 Sims CA, Wattanasirichaigoon S, Menconi MJ, Ajami AM, Fink MP. Ringer's ethyl pyruvate solution ameliorates ischemia/reperfusion-induced intestinal mucosal injury in rats. *Crit Care Med* 2001;**29**:1513–18.
20 Åneman A, Pettersson A, Eisenhofer G, *et al*. Sympathetic and renin-angiotensis activation during graded hypovolemia in pigs: Impact on mesenteric perfusion and duodenal mucosal function. *Shock* 1997;**8**:378–84.
21 Von Ritter C, Grisham MB, Hollwarth M, Inauen W, Granger DN. Neutrophil-derived oxidants mediate formyl-methionyl-leucyl-phenylalanine-induced increases in mucosal permeability in rats. *Gastroenterology* 1989;**3**:778–80.
22 Xia ZF, Hollyoak M, Barrow RE, He F, Muller MJ, Herndon DN. Superoxide dismutase and leupeptin prevent delayed reperfusion injury in the small intestine during burn shock. *J Burn Care Rehabil* 1995;**16**:111–17.
23 Cicalese L, Lee K, Schraut W, Watkins S, Borle A, Stanko R. Pyruvate prevents ischemia-reperfusion mucosal injury of rat small intestine. *Am J Surg* 1996;**171**:97–100.
24 Schleiffer R, Raul F. Prophylactic administration of L-arginine improves the intestinal barrier function after mesenteric ischaemia. *Gut* 1996;**39**:94–8.

6: Medical management of non-variceal upper gastrointestinal haemorrhage

PAUL WINWOOD

Introduction

Acute upper gastrointestinal (GI) haemorrhage is a relatively common reason for admission to hospital and until recently there has been little change in mortality over the last fifty years. Acute GI bleeding also occurs in patients already in hospital and contributes significantly to overall mortality. Critically ill patients in particular are at increased risk of developing bleeding in the upper GI tract, usually as a result of peptic ulceration. Most patients with acute upper GI haemorrhage are managed conservatively or with endoscopic intervention but some ultimately require surgery to arrest the haemorrhage. Endoscopic therapy has become a mainstay in the management of upper GI haemorrhage and this is the area in which there has been perhaps the most advances in the last decade. This article describes the incidence and risk of re-bleeding and mortality in patients with bleeding ulcers, and describes available therapeutic options.

Epidemiology of upper gastrointestinal bleeding

Current knowledge of the epidemiology of upper GI haemorrhage is scanty. In the few population based studies undertaken in the United Kingdom, reported incidence varies from 47 per 100 000 to 116 per 100 000, with overall mortality approximately 10%.[1,2] In the elderly the incidence is much higher at around 475 per 100 000.[2] Upper GI bleeding is an important cause of emergency admission to hospital accounting for about 8% of admissions. The incidence of upper GI haemorrhage in patients who are already in hospital is also significant and these patients have the highest mortality, especially in the critically ill.[3]

Mortality figures over the last 50 or so years are, on first inspection, disappointing. Data from acute admissions due to GI bleeding from the 1940s indicates mortality of around 10% which remained constant even in the 1960s and 1990s. However the percentage of elderly patients has increased dramatically, and in fact age-standardised mortality has decreased (Table 6.1).[2] Bleeding from ulcers ceases spontaneously in at least 80% of patients most of whom have an uneventful recovery without a specific intervention. However, the sub-group of patients with upper GI bleeding who do not do well, accounts for the overall mortality rate. There are two possible explanations for the unchanging mortality rate. Firstly, age and the prevalence of concurrent illness continue to rise among patients presenting with upper GI bleeding. Patients with bleeding usually die not from exsanguination but from decompensation due to other diseases. Secondly, until very recently, effective non-surgical methods for the control of bleeding from ulcers were not available.

Table 6.1 Mortality from upper gastrointestinal bleeding.

Reference	Mortality %	Age standardised mortality %2
Jones[4] 1940–47	9·9	147
Johnston et al.[5] 1967–8	10·6	122
Rockall et al.[2] 1993	11·3	100

In 1995, Rockall and colleagues reported a large study to describe the epidemiology of acute upper GI haemorrhage in the UK. Over a four-month period, 4 185 cases of acute upper GI haemorrhage were documented.[2] The overall incidence of acute upper GI haemorrhage was 103/100 000 adults per year and the incidence rose from 23/100 000 in people less than 30 years old to 485/100 000 in those aged over 75. The incidence in men was double that in women except in elderly patients. Fourteen per cent occurred in in-patients. Overall mortality was 14% (11% in emergency admissions and 33% in inpatients). It was concluded that the incidence of acute upper GI haemorrhage increases appreciably with age and that deaths occurred almost exclusively in very old patients or those with severe co-morbidity.

A more recent study published in 2000 investigated upper GI haemorrhage which developed while in hospital, in patients on ICU.[6] Peptic ulcer disease was present in 56% of patients and was the most common source of bleeding identified. The in-hospital mortality rate was 42% and the cause of death was sepsis and/or multiple system organ failure in 75% of patients. No patients died directly as a result of GI bleeding.

In dedicated GI bleeding units, mortality rates as a direct consequence of bleeding are reported to be as low as 2%. A study of 701 patients with bleeding peptic ulcers reported a mortality rate of 10% in patients over the age of 60 years, compared with only 0·5% in those who were 60 or younger.[7] In this author's experience, the introduction of a GI bleeding protocol resulted in a reduction of mortality to 8·9%, despite a predominantly elderly population, with a mean age of around 70 years (Figure 6.1). Ideally, mortality in patients under 60 years should be zero, and certainly less than 0·5%.

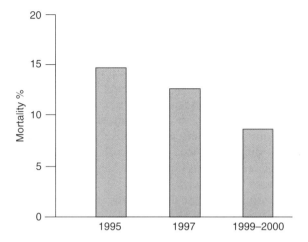

Figure 6.1 Mortality in patients with upper gastrointestinal bleeding presenting to the Gastroenterology Unit at the Royal Bournemouth Hospital between 1995 and 2000 following the introduction of a protocol in 1995. The mean age of these patients was 70 years.

Patients on ICU

Studies of patients admitted to intensive care units (ICU) have reported overt bleeding in up to a third of patients and endoscopically identifiable mucosal abnormalities in up to 100% of patients. The variation in the reported frequency of development of GI bleeding in severely ill patients probably reflects different definitions of clinical bleeding and varying practice in terms of prophylactic therapy. Gastrointestinal bleeding has an associated mortality of 20–40% in hospitalized patients. Respiratory failure, hypotension, coagulopathy and sepsis have been identified as risk factors for upper GI bleeding in critically ill patients. Studies have also shown that mechanical ventilation is a strong risk factor for nosocomial GI bleeding, in addition to administration of total parenteral nutrition, prior organ transplant, and malignancy.

Origin of upper gastrointestinal bleeding

Peptic ulcers are the most common cause of serious upper GI bleeding. Approximately 50% of upper GI bleeding is due to peptic ulcers. Other causes include oesophageal erosions, Mallory-Weiss tears and oesophageal varices. Eighty per cent of uncomplicated peptic ulcers stop bleeding spontaneously, but 20% either continue bleeding or the patient dies. It is clearly important to have some means of assessing firstly who is at risk of GI bleeding and secondly, having bled, some means of assessing the risk of continued bleeding or death.

Pre-disposition to bleeding from ulcers

The two factors which have the most impact on risk of bleeding from peptic ulcers are age and non-steroidal anti-inflammatory drug (NSAID) usage. Over the age of 60 years the risk of GI bleed increases three fold. Perhaps surprisingly, increased acid secretion is not associated with bleeding in patients with peptic ulcers. It has been shown that both basal and stimulated acid output and parietal cell sensitivity to pentagastrin is similar in patients with duodenal ulcers whether they are bleeding or not. The prevalence of *Helicobacter pylori* infection is also unrelated to haemorrhage of ulcers. However, the use of NSAIDs is an important risk factor. A number of large studies suggest that the risk of upper GI bleeding is higher in patients who use NSAIDs than in those who do not. Indeed a meta-analysis found that in patients over 60 years, the use of NSAIDs for less than one month was associated with higher risks of complications.[8] Ingestion of NSAIDs may cause both gastric and duodenal ulcers such that NSAIDs not only induce ulcers but also increase the chance of bleeding in patients whose underlying ulcer disease is not primarily due to these drugs.

Aspirin also increases the risk of an ulcer bleeding. The risk of bleeding was assessed in a large randomised controlled trial of aspirin therapy for prophylaxis against transient ischaemic attacks.[9] Patients received either 300 or 1200 mg aspirin a day or placebo. Patients receiving 300 mg of aspirin had a significant increase in upper GI bleeding, compared with those receiving placebo, and in those patients receiving 1 200 mg/day aspirin the relative risk of bleeding was twice that for the patients receiving the lower dose. Corticosteroids alone probably do not increase the risk of ulcer development or bleeding, but have been reported to double the NSAID-associated risk of serious GI complications,[8] and the combined use of steroids and NSAIDs have been shown to be associated with a 10-fold increase in the risk of upper GI bleeding.[10] A recent paper, however, suggest that corticosteriods do cause ulcers and GI bleeding even without other risk factors.[11] Although anticoagulation therapy may be thought to increase the risk of bleeding in patients with peptic ulcers, reports suggest that patients treated with anticoagulants have a similar incidence of ulcer haemorrhage as other patients.[12]

Clinical presentation and prognostic indicators

About 20% of patients who have bleeding ulcers present with melaena, 30% with haematemesis, and 50% with both.[13] As many as 5% present with haematochezia. A number of end points for assessment of patients with bleeding ulcers have been used, including number of units of blood transfused, requirements for urgent surgery, and mortality. Contributory factors to these criteria include the severity of the first bleed, whether re-bleeding occurs, and the age and co-morbidity of the patient.

Table 6.2 Ulcer appearance at endoscopy and re-bleeding and mortality.

Appearance at endoscopy	Re-bleeding %	Mortality %
Clean base	5	2
Flat spot	10	3
Adherent clot	22	7
Non-bleeding visible vessel	43	11
Actively bleeding	55	11

Data are from prospective trials where patients did not receive endoscopic therapy.[13]

Endoscopic stigmata for the assessment of risk of re-bleeding

Clearly clinical characteristics are important in predicting the outcome from an upper GI bleed, and enable determination of which patients should undergo urgent endoscopy, but the endoscopic appearance of a bleeding ulcer also provides useful prognostic information (Table 6.2).[14] The appearance of the ulcer in terms of stigmata of haemorrhage, for example, the presence of clots or active spurting, has a direct association with the risk of re-bleeding. The size of an ulcer is also a prognostic indicator – large ulcers (>2 cm) are linked with increased rates of re-bleeding and death, even after endoscopic haemostatic therapy. A small study also reported that the endoscopic appearance of vessels is associated with risk of re-bleeding, such that clear or translucent vessels presage a significantly higher likelihood of re-bleeding than more opaque vessels.[15] Blood flow beneath the surface of the ulcer, measured using a Doppler probe passed through the biopsy channel of an endoscope has been used as a prognostic indicator. Re-bleeding seems to be rare when no blood flow is detected by Doppler.[16]

Risk factors for mortality

A simple numerical scoring system has been developed from the Rockall epidemiological study (described above) which enables rational categorisation of mortality risk in patients with upper GI haemorrhage.[17] A prospective, unselected, multicentre, population based study was undertaken using standardized questionnaires in two phases one year apart. A total of 4 185 cases of acute upper GI haemorrhage over the age of 16 identified over a four-month period in 1993[2] and 1 625 cases identified subsequently over a three-month period in 1994 were included in the study.[17] It was found that age, shock, co-morbidity, diagnosis, major stigmata of recent haemorrhage, and re-bleeding are all independent predictors of mortality when assessed using multiple logistic regression. A numerical score using these parameters was developed (Table 6.3). When tested for general applicability in a second population, the scoring system was found to reproducibly predict mortality in each risk category. This simple numerical score (the "Rockall" score) can be used to categorise patients presenting with acute upper GI haemorrhage by risk of death. This score can be used to determine case mix when comparing outcomes in audit and research and to calculate risk standardized mortality. In addition, this score can identify 15% of all cases with acute upper GI haemorrhage at the time of presentation and 26% of cases after endoscopy who are at low risk of re-bleeding and negligible risk of death and who might therefore be considered for early discharge or outpatient treatment. The Rockall score provides an initial score based on clinical presentation and a second score after endoscopy. Mortality increases with the increase in score (Figure 6.2).

Table 6.3 Contributors to the Rockall score.[18]

Contributor	Score			
	0	1	2	3
Age	<60	60–79	>80	
Shock	None	Pulse < 100 BP > 100	BP > 100	
Co-morbidity	None		CCF/IHD or other	Renal/liver failure, disseminated malignancy
Diagnosis	None or Mallory Weiss	All others	Upper GI tract malignancy	
Endoscopic stigmata	None		Blood in upper GI tract/adherent clot/visible vessel	

CCF – congestive cardiac failure
IHD – ischaemic heart disease

The Rockall score can also be used to assist in the management of patients with upper GI bleeding. In this author's unit, if the initial score (based on clinical criteria) is >3 central venous pressure is monitored; if the total score after endoscopy is >5 there should be joint management

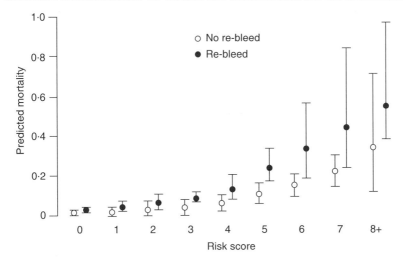

Figure 6.2 Plot of computer predicted mortality by risk score (median and range) showing the degree of association between the predictions of the model and the observed mortality for each score. See text for details. Redrawn from Rockall TA, et al. Gut 1996;38:316–21[17] with permission from the BMJ Publishing Group.

with the upper GI surgical team; finally if the total score is 0–1 patients are discharged after 24 hours.

It is possible, however, to rely too heavily on scoring systems and protocols which should be used only to guide clinical practice. Immediate endoscopic or surgical assessment is recommended for anyone with continuing shock, defined as systolic blood pressure less than 100 mmHg, anyone who is over 60 years who has had more than 4 units of blood transfused and anyone who has had more than 8 units. Patients with a systolic blood pressure of <80 mmHg should be referred immediately to the GI unit for consideration for surgery.

Strategies for management

Medical management of upper GI bleeding begins initially with resuscitation, depending on the amount of blood loss and the patient's clinical condition. Haemodynamic assessment (blood pressure, pulse, and postural changes) and, if necessary, institution of resuscitative measures are the first steps in the management of upper GI bleeding (Box 6.1). The next important step in the process is to evaluate risk, including both risk of re-bleeding and risk of mortality. Early diagnosis through endoscopy enables effective action according to the perceived risk. This should be undertaken within 12 and no more than 24 hours after haemorrhage or admission. Throughout this process it is important to monitor the patient and intervene as appropriate.

Box 6.1 Management strategies for upper gastrointestinal bleeding

- Resuscitation
- Evaluation of risk
- Endoscopy within 24 hours
- Monitoring
- Referral for surgery or endoscopic therapy

In terms of management, endoscopic therapy is preferred in the first instance. Department of Health guidelines state that every hospital managing upper GI haemorrhage should have therapeutic endoscopy available 24 hours a day. Overall, 5% of patients with upper GI haemorrhage have surgery although the surgical intervention rate is up to four times higher in patients with upper GI bleed admitted to surgical units than for those admitted under medical teams.[19] In patients with acute upper GI haemorrhage surgical intervention is largely confined to the highest-risk patients and the continuing high mortality in such patients is therefore to be expected. As endoscopic therapy becomes the first line of treatment for high risk patients, the mortality rate should decrease.

Therapeutic options

Endoscopy is widely used to evaluate and treat GI haemorrhage. This may include patients with bleeding at admission or critically ill patients whose bleeding develops while in the hospital.

Endoscopic therapy

The lack of any clearly effective medical therapy for patients with bleeding ulcers has prompted a search for alternative forms of haemostatic therapy. The development of a variety of endoscopic therapies, shown in Box 6.2, is the most important advance in the treatment of bleeding ulcers over the past decade.

In studies with animals, laser therapy is less effective than the other thermal devices. Controlled trials of argon and neodymium-yttrium-aluminium-garnet lasers have yielded mixed results, although in the meta-analysis by Cook *et al.* it was revealed that laser therapy did significantly reduce the rates of further bleeding, urgent surgery, and mortality.[20] However, it is possible to cause transmural injury using laser and this

---

Box 6.2 Options for endoscopic therapy

- Thermal
    Electrocoagulation
    Heater probe
    Laser
- Injection
    Epinephrine
    Sclerosants
    Ethanol
    Thrombin
    Fibrin Glue
- Mechanical
    Haemoclip
    Staple
    Suture

---

therapy thus requires a high degree of technical expertise (in addition to its high cost compared to other techniques).

Monopolar electrocoagulation, bipolar electrocoagulation, and heater-probe therapy use thermal contact to cause haemostasis. Monopolar electrocoagulation has been replaced by the other two methods primarily since monopolar electrocoagulation causes more tissue injury. Prospective, randomized trials have demonstrated that these approaches result in a significant reduction in re-bleeding, the requirement for blood transfusions, the length of hospital stay, and the need for urgent surgery in patients with clinical evidence of major bleeding and endoscopic evidence of actively bleeding ulcers or non-bleeding ulcers with visible vessels.[21] In 1989 a National Institutes of Health consensus conference recommended bipolar electrocoagulation and heater-probe therapy in the approach to endoscopic haemostasis.

Injection therapy is a non-thermal method of inducing haemostasis. Solutions including ethanol, epinephrine or sclerosing agents are injected into the base of the ulcer with a catheter that has a retractable needle. The fact that normal saline is also effective suggests that at least one mechanism of haemostasis is simply local compression of the blood vessel by the injected solution. Whether the addition of a sclerosant after epinephrine or saline injection is better than either alone is unclear. However, Chung *et al.* compared endoscopic epinephrine injection alone and epinephrine injection plus heater probe in the management of 276 patients with actively bleeding ulcers detected by endoscopy within 24 hours of admission.[22] Patients were randomised to either endoscopic epinephrine injection alone (n=136) or epinephrine injection plus heater probe treatment (n=140). Initial haemostasis was achieved in 98% who received epinephrine injection alone and 99% who received additional heater probe treatment. Outcome as measured by clinical re-bleeding, requirement for emergency operation, blood transfusion, hospital stay, ulcer healing at four weeks, and in-hospital mortality were not significantly different in the two groups. In the subgroup of patients with spurting haemorrhage the relative risk of surgical intervention was lower in the dual treatment group. Therefore, heater-probe treatment after endoscopic epinephrine injection may offer an advantage in ulcers with spurting haemorrhage.

Mechanical methods used include suturing, clipping or stapling the bleeding ulcer, but these techniques are generally less effective than either injection or bipolar electrocoagulation and heater-probe therapy.

Most trials of endoscopic therapy have been able to report a significant reduction in mortality. Meta-analyses have described a lower mortality in patients receiving endoscopic treatment for upper GI bleeding, compared with those not receiving such therapy.[20,23,24]

The two major complications of endoscopic therapy, perforation and uncontrollable bleeding, are, fortunately, rare. Endoscopic therapy is not required in most patients with bleeding ulcers, only in those with clinical evidence of substantial bleeding (for example, haemodynamic instability with tachycardia, hypotension, or postural changes in blood pressure or pulse; a dropping haematocrit; or the need for transfusions) and endoscopic evidence of active bleeding or a non-bleeding visible vessel. As highlighted in Table 6.2, in ulcers with a flat spot or clean base, bleeding recurs much less commonly and these do not benefit from endoscopic therapy. Most authorities advise endoscopic therapy for ulcers with adherent clot, but this is controversial since the rebleeding rate and mortality are still relatively low in this situation (22% and 7% respectively) and therapeutic intervention carries the risk of precipitating further bleeding.

It is unclear whether re-bleeding after therapeutic endoscopy should lead to surgery or further endoscopic therapy. Re-bleeding of peptic ulcers occurs in 15 to 20% of patients. Lau et al.[25] compared endoscopic re-treatment with surgery after initial endoscopy in patients with recurrent bleeding; 48 patients were randomly assigned to undergo immediate endoscopic re-treatment and 44 were assigned to undergo surgery. Thirty five (73%) of those treated with repeat endoscopy did not require surgery and there was a non-significant lower mortality in the endoscopic retreatment group (5 of 48 compared with 8 of 47). There were also fewer complications than with surgery. Repeated treatment can thus be attempted in patients with recurrent bleeding. Patients who are going to fail with endoscopic therapy can be predicted at endoscopy to some extent, for example large posterior wall duodenal ulcers and high lesser curve ulcers with visible vessels. Also, there is undoubtedly a window of opportunity when the chances of surviving surgery are at their best. The decision to repeat endoscopic therapy against surgery needs to be considered carefully in the context of the patient's co-morbidity and likely clinical course if they have further hypotensive bleeding episodes.

Surgery

Surgery is generally performed for continued haemorrhage or rebleeding when endoscopic therapy has failed or is unavailable. For the patient with rapid haemorrhage and haemodynamic instability who cannot be controlled endoscopically, operation is clearly indicated. For patients with a moderate risk of recurrent ulcer haemorrhage, the clinician must make a decision based on what is known of the clinical and endoscopic predictors of recurrent haemorrhage regarding the selective use of endoscopic haemostasis and early operation. For elderly patients with a large ulcer who have had significant blood loss resulting in hypovolaemic shock, and who have endoscopic stigmata of ulcer haemorrhage, early elective operation after endoscopic haemostasis may be the most judicious course. Surgery may also be a wise choice for those patients in whom an initially successful attempt at endoscopic haemostasis fails, especially if there are predictive factors for failure of endoscopic therapy.

Recommendations for the surgical management of bleeding ulcers include immediate operation for patients who are rapidly exsanguinating and patients who are active bleeding despite attempts at endoscopic haemostasis. In addition early elective operation after initial endoscopic haemostasis for elderly patients with co-morbid disease and/or haemodynamic instability who have active arterial ulcer haemorrhage controlled with endoscopic haemostasis, should be considered. In elderly patients with co-morbid disease and/or haemodynamic instability who have a visible vessel in an ulcer crater treated with endoscopic haemostasis, surgery is advised, particularly for those with a positive arterial Doppler signal in the ulcer crater, a large posterior duodenal ulcer or a large high lesser-curvature gastric ulcer. Surgery is also advised for elderly patients with co-morbid disease and/or haemodynamic instability who develop recurrent ulcer bleeding while hospitalised or who have a requirement for blood transfusion of 5 or more units.

Angiographic therapy

Angiographic therapy is rarely used to treat patients with bleeding ulcers and should be considered only for severe, persistent bleeding if surgery poses an extremely high risk and endoscopic therapy has been unsuccessful

63

or is unavailable. Ulcers may stop bleeding with an intra-arterial infusion of vasopressin in about half of cases.[26] Uncontrolled studies suggest that arterial embolisation with an absorbable gelatine sponge, an autologous clot, tissue adhesives, or mechanical occlusion devices may control bleeding identified angiographically in some cases. Recurrent bleeding, ischaemia with stenosis, infarction, perforation, or abscesses have been reported following embolisation therapy.[14,27]

Prophylaxis for recurrent bleeding

The ultimate goal in preventing recurrent bleeding is successful healing of the ulcer. Bleeding and non-bleeding ulcers heal at the same rates following haemostasis.[28] Although follow-up endoscopy may be required to rule out cancer in upper GI bleeding and for some high risk cases, routine repeat endoscopy to document healing is not necessary, although maximisation of healing by higher doses or longer courses of anti-secretory therapy may be warranted, particularly with large ulcers.

In a study by Jensen and co-workers,[29] a 36% incidence of re-bleeding in patients who had a bleeding duodenal ulcer was reported, indicating the importance of eliminating as many risk factors for recurrence as possible for an individual patient. These include the use of NSAIDs, infection with *H. pylori*, and gastric acid.

Pharmacological approaches

There is no convincing evidence that gastric lavage with any fluid at any temperature will stop bleeding or prevent recurrent bleeding.[30] Pharmacological agents which act through vasoconstriction or reduce gastric acidity or both, including vasopressin, secretin, prostaglandins, somatostatin, and H_2-receptor antagonists, have been used in an attempt to induce haemostasis in actively bleeding ulcers. Although a few studies have reported some benefit, on the whole these agents are ineffective.[31-34]

Data from *in vitro* studies have suggested that clotting is more effective and proteolytic degradation of clots occurs more slowly at high pH,[33] such that reduction of gastric acidity may delay re-bleeding. However, in randomized, placebo-controlled trials of histamine-2 (H2)-receptor antagonists, omeprazole, somatostatin or prostaglandins there was no reduction in the incidence of re-bleeding even when combined with antacids to maintain gastric pH at 7·0.[31,34,35] A recent study has shown a reduced re-bleeding rate with intravenous omeprazole after endoscopic therapy of bleeding peptic ulcers[36] but further studies are required.

Tranexamic acid, which inhibits fibrinolysis, has also been used to promote clot formation. A meta-analysis of six controlled trials of tranexamic acid showed no statistically significant reduction in recurrent bleeding or the need for surgery but overall mortality was decreased.[37] However, these trials were not confined to bleeding ulcers and as such the applicability of these results to the management of bleeding ulcers is uncertain. Tranexamic acid is not approved for the treatment of bleeding ulcers in the UK.

Obscure GI bleeding may be further investigated with colonoscopy, enteroscopy and angiography, applying endoscopic haemostasis and embolisation respectively when required.

Conclusions

Acute upper gastrointestinal bleeding is a common reason for hospitalisation and also commonly occurs in critically ill patients already on the ICU. Overall, mortality rates range from 5% to 15%; patients with severe co-morbidities and those with persistent or recurrent bleeding are at highest risk. Accurate preliminary risk assessment and resuscitation should proceed simultaneously at initial presentation. Risk assessment can guide treatment decisions. Early upper GI endoscopy, a cornerstone of management, allows for rapid diagnosis, application of endoscopic therapy, and completion of risk assessment. Endoscopic therapy can alter the natural history of upper GI bleeding by reducing rates of further bleeding and, consequently, mortality. Complete risk assessment of both clinical and endoscopic factors may also result in shorter hospital stays and other improved outcomes. Limited data are available concerning the endoscopic findings and the effectiveness of endoscopic therapy versus surgery in reducing mortality in severely ill patients with bleeding that develops while in the hospital or the ICU. Critical care doctors must therefore make recommendations for their patients by extrapolating results of studies of patients admitted for bleeding. Because the mortality rate is so high in this population, better knowledge of the probability of finding a lesion amenable to endoscopic therapy can help clinicians decide which therapeutic option is most appropriate.

References

1 Berry AR, Collin J, Frostick SP, Dudley NE, Morris PJ. Upper gastrointestinal haemorrhage in Oxford. *J R Coll Surg Edinb* 1984;**29**:134–8.
2 Rockall TA, Logan RF, Devlin HB, Northfield TC. Incidence of and mortality from acute upper gastrointestinal haemorrhage in the United Kingdom. Steering Committee and members of the National Audit of Acute Upper Gastrointestinal Haemorrhage. *BMJ* 1995;**311**:222–6.
3 Terdiman JP, Ostroff JW. Gastrointestinal bleeding in the hospitalized patient: a case-control study to assess risk factors, causes, and outcome. *Am J Med* 1998;**104**:349–54.
4 Jones FA. Haematemesis and melaena with special reference to bleeding peptic ulcer. *BMJ* 1947;**ii**:441–6.

5 Johnston SJ, Jones PF, Kyle J, Needham CD. Epidemiology and course of gastrointestinal haemorrhage in north-east Scotland. *BMJ* 1973;**iii**:655–60.

6 Lewis JD, Shin EJ, Metz DC. Characterization of gastrointestinal bleeding in severely ill hospitalized patients. *Crit Care Med* 2000;**28**:46–50.

7 Branicki FJ, Coleman SY, Fok PJ, *et al.* Bleeding peptic ulcer: a prospective evaluation of risk factors for rebleeding and mortality. *World J Surg* 1990;**14**: 262–70.

8 Gabriel SE, Jaakkimainen L, Bombardier C. Risk for serious gastrointestinal complications related to use of nonsteroidal anti-inflammatory drugs: a meta-analysis. *Ann Intern Med* 1991;**115**:787–96.

9 Shorrock CJ, Langman MJS, Warlow C. Risks of upper GI bleeding during TIA prophylaxis with aspirin. *Gastroenterology* 1992;**102**:A165.

10 Piper JM, Ray WA, Daugherty JR, Griffin MR. Corticosteroid use and peptic ulcer disease: role of nonsteroidal anti-inflammatory drugs. *Ann Intern Med* 1991;**114**:735–40.

11 Nielsen GL, Sorensen HT, Mellemkjoer L, *et al.* Risk of hospitalization resulting from upper gastroinstestinal bleeding among patients taking corticosteroids: a register based cohort study. *Am J Med* 2001;**111**:541–5.

12 Choudari CP, Rajgopal C, Palmer KR. Acute gastrointestinal haemorrhage in anticoagulated patients: diagnoses and response to endoscopic treatment. *Gut* 1994;**35**:464–6.

13 Wara P, Stodkilde H. Bleeding pattern before admission as guideline for emergency endoscopy. *Scand J Gastroenterol* 1985;**20**:72–8.

14 Laine L, Peterson WL. Bleeding peptic ulcer. *N Engl J Med* 1994;**331**:717–27.

15 Freeman ML, Cass OW, Peine CJ, Onstad GR. The non-bleeding visible vessel versus the sentinel clot: natural history and risk of rebleeding. *Gastrointest Endosc* 1993;**39**:359–66.

16 Fullarton GM, Murray WR. Prediction of rebleeding in peptic ulcers by visual stigmata and endoscopic Doppler ultrasound criteria. *Endoscopy* 1990;**22**:68–71.

17 Rockall TA, Logan RF, Devlin HB, Northfield TC. Risk assessment after acute upper gastrointestinal haemorrhage. *Gut* 1996;**38**:316–21.

18 Rockall TA. Acute upper gastrointestinal haemorrhage. *Gastroenterol Hepatol Nutr* 1999;**2**:72–4.

19 Cochran TA. Bleeding peptic ulcer: surgical therapy. *Gastroenterol Clin North Am* 1993;**22**:751–78.

20 Cook DJ, Guyatt GH, Salena BJ, Laine LA. Endoscopic therapy for acute nonvariceal upper gastrointestinal hemorrhage: a meta-analysis. *Gastroenterology* 1992;**102**:139–48.

21 Allan R, Dykes P. A study of the factors influencing mortality rates from gastrointestinal haemorrhage. *Q J Med* 1976;**45**:533–50.

22 Chung SS, Lau JY, Sung JJ, *et al.* Randomised comparison between adrenaline injection alone and adrenaline injection plus heat probe treatment for actively bleeding ulcers. *BMJ* 1997;**314**:1307–11.

23 Laine L, Cook D. Endoscopic ligation compared with sclerotherapy for treatment of esophageal variceal bleeding. A meta-analysis. *Ann Intern Med* 1995;**123**:280–7.

24 Sacks HS, Chalmers TC, Blum AL, Berrier J, Pagano D. Endoscopic hemostasis: an effective therapy for bleeding peptic ulcers. *J Am Med Assoc* 1990;**264**:494–9.

25 Lau JY, Sung JJ, Lam YH, *et al.* Endoscopic retreatment compared with surgery in patients with recurrent bleeding after initial endoscopic control of bleeding ulcers. *N Engl J Med* 1999;**340**:751–6.

26 Sherman LM, Shenoy SS, Cerra FB. Selective intra-arterial vasopressin: clinical efficacy and complications. *Ann Surg* 1979;**189**:298–302.

27 Lang EK. Transcatheter embolization in management of hemorrhage from duodenal ulcer: long-term results and complications. *Radiology* 1992;**182**:703–7.

28 Murray WR, Laferla G, Cooper G, Archibald M. Duodenal ulcer healing after presentation with haemorrhage. *Gut* 1986;**27**:1387–9.

29 Jensen DM, Cheng S, Kovacs TOG, *et al.* A controlled study of ranitidine for the prevention of recurrent hemorrhage from duodenal ulcer. *N Engl J Med* 1994;**330**:382–6.

30 Ponsky JL, Hoffman M, Swayngim DS. Saline irrigation in gastric hemorrhage: the effect of temperature. *J Surg Res* 1980;**28**:204–5.

31 Zuckerman G, Welch R, Douglas A, *et al.* Controlled trial of medical therapy for active upper gastrointestinal bleeding and prevention of rebleeding. *Am J Med* 1984;**76**:361–6.

32 Magnusson I, Ihre T, Johansson C, Seligson U, Torngren S, Uvnas-Moberg K. Randomised double blind trial of somatostatin in the treatment of massive upper gastrointestinal haemorrhage. *Gut* 1985;**26**:221–6.

33 Patchett SE, Enright H, Afdhal N, O'Connell W, O'Donoghue DP. Clot lysis by gastric juice: an *in vitro* study. *Gut* 1989;**30**:1704–7.

34 Daneshmend TK, Hawkey CJ, Langman MJS, Logan RFA, Long RG, Walt RP. Omeprazole versus placebo for acute upper gastrointestinal bleeding: randomised double blind controlled trial. *BMJ* 1992;**304**:143–7.

35 Walt RP, Cottrell J, Mann SG, Freemantle NP, Langman MJS. Continuous intravenous famotidine for haemorrhage from peptic ulcer. *Lancet* 1992;**340**:1058–62.

36 Lau JY, Sung JJ, Lee KK, *et al.* Effect of intravenous omeprazole on recurrent bleeding after endoscopic treatment of bleeding peptic ulcers. *New Engl J Med* 2000;**343**:310–16.

37 Henry DA, O'Connell DL. Effects of fibrinolytic inhibitors on mortality from upper gastrointestinal haemorrhage. *BMJ* 1989;**298**:1142–6.

7: Acute pancreatitis

JOHN R CLARK, JANE EDDLESTON

Introduction

Acute pancreatitis is a common disease on the intensive care unit, which is ruled by its complications, despite considerable increases in knowledge (as a result of animal studies) concerning the seminal events within the pancreatic acinar cell at the evolution of the acute inflammation. This article describes the epidemiology, aetiology and controversial clinical issues including feeding, new therapies and thoughts on future therapeutic options.

Initial events

Irrespective of the putative aetiological agent or its route of attack, breakdown in the regulated secretory pathway towards exocytosis in the acinar cell appears always to be the initiating event. It is now generally accepted that this breakdown of normal signal transduction can be attributed to a burst of free radical activity within the cell, outstripping endogenous antioxidant defences,[1] and resulting in "pancreastasis".[2] The physiological response is deft. The bulk of secretions are diverted into the interstitium by the vesicular pathway in the basolateral membrane[3] to be drained away by lymphatics and the bloodstream. This is seen diagnostically as an early rise in the activity of pancreatic enzymes in blood and urine.[4,5] In addition, the intracellular lysosomal and zymogen granule compartments coalesce to enable excess zymogen to be "detonated" safely and then removed. This reversal in secretory polarity and secretory diversion is the basis for the ensuing inflammatory response. So powerful is the inflammatory response that the term "frustrated phagocytosis" has been coined.[6] Since pancreatic secretions are not inflammatory *per se*, lipid and protein oxidation fragments and cytokines, such as platelet-activating factor (PAF) produced by the injured acinar cell, are a more plausible trigger for the response. The speed and the intensity of the systemic

68

inflammatory response which accompanies the acute pancreatic inflammation is swift and continues to thwart many innovative therapies.

Epidemiology

Acute pancreatitis has an incidence of 30–50 per 1 00 000 of the population and produces a spectrum of symptoms, which range from mild and self-limiting to severe necrosis of the pancreas resulting in acute necrotising pancreatitis (ANP) and multi-organ dysfunction. It has been estimated that one in four patients with acute pancreatitis will have a severe attack and one in four of this sub-group will die as a result. This translates into an overall death rate of 6% but in reality the mortality is considerably higher, reported to be about 20% in a recent large-scale study.[7] Within the sub-population of ANP the mortality may be as high as 45%.[8] The majority of deaths (60%) will occur within the first three weeks, whilst later deaths usually represent a subsequent infective complication.

Aetiology

The aetiology of pancreatitis can be broadly classified as primary or that resulting from critical illness due to another underlying cause. With an increased awareness of this latter group, the incidence of pancreatic dysfunction is increasing.

The majority of primary cases (approximately 70%) are accounted for by biliary stones and/or alcohol abuse. Acute idiopathic pancreatitis occurs in approximately 20–40% of cases, although biliary sludge can be demonstrated in many instances. A minority (5–10%) of cases are caused by a variety of other conditions listed in Box 7.1. The exact nature of the aetiological factor has an important bearing on prognosis, investigations and management of these patients.

Increasingly it is being recognised that pancreatic dysfunction can occur in any critically ill patient and the clinical consequence of this can range from the infrequent but often-fatal necrotising pancreatitis to the more common sub-clinical hyperamylasaemia. The mechanism of such pancreatic dysfunction is likely to be multifaceted. Potential factors include ischaemia/reperfusion injury and circulating factors.

Ischaemia and reperfusion

Animal models of shock have consistently demonstrated impairment of pancreatic blood flow. In a rat model of ischaemia-reperfusion following clamping of splanchnic vessels, a significant reduction of functional

69

Box 7.1 Aetiology of acute primary pancreatitis

Percentage   *Cause*

- 70%   Biliary stones (more common in females)
            Alcohol abuse (more common in males)

- 20–40%   Idiopathic

- 5–10%   Post-operative or post-endoscopic retrograde
              cholangiography
            Abdominal trauma
            Drugs – metronidazole, valproate, azathioprine,
              steroids, diuretics
            Viral infections – hepatitis, cytomegalo virus, mumps
            Hypertriglyceridaemia
            Hypercalcaemia
            Systemic vasculitis
            Tumours
            Inherited or acquired abnormalities of pancreatic
              ducts or papilla

---

capillary density within the pancreas was observed.[9] Post-ischaemic reperfusion was also associated with an increase in serum lipase and histological alterations, characterised by interstitial oedema and a diffuse inflammatory response.[9]

More pronounced impairment of the pancreatic blood flow compared to other regional and systemic flows seems to occur in shock. In a pig model of acute haemorrhage and reperfusion, the blood flow to the pancreas decreased significantly more than in the other splanchnic regions, suggesting that the pancreas is particularly vulnerable to haemorrhage.[10] A disproportionate decrease in pancreatic blood flow was also reported in a pig model of cardiogenic shock after pericardial tamponade.[11] Impaired pancreatic perfusion has also been found in animal models of sepsis, with reduced blood flow occurring independently of changes in systemic perfusion pressures.[12,13] Other work also supports the concept that blood flow is preferentially redistributed away from the pancreas in sepsis.[14–16]

Impaired splanchnic circulation could also arise from the application of high-pressure positive end-expiratory pressure (PEEP). Histological evidence that pancreatic acinar cell injury and an increase in serum amylase and lipase activity occurs with high levels of PEEP has been reported in a pig model and similar effects on splanchnic blood flow have been reported in acute respiratory distress syndrome (ARDS) patients.[17] Furthermore in man, increases in circulating pancreatic enzyme activity following aortic cross-clamping or cardiopulmonary bypass have been shown to correlate with reductions in pancreatic blood flow.[18,19]

Circulating factors

Circulating factors may exert an effect on pancreatic function by influencing pancreatic blood flow or acinar function. Somatostatin is a regulatory peptide, produced by neuroendocrine, inflammatory and immune cells. It is released in large amounts from storage pools of secretory cells or in small amounts from activated immune and inflammatory cells. It acts as an endogenous inhibitory regulator of the secretory and proliferative responses of widely distributed target cells. Somatostatin has been found to decrease gastric, duodenal, jejunal and pancreatic blood flow, and to reduce pancreatic enzyme and bicarbonate output. It also has an inhibitory affect on gastrointestinal motility.[20]

In animal experiments, an increase in serum somatostatin occurs in cardiogenic,[21] haemorrhagic[22] and endotoxic shock,[23,24] as well as in endogenous peritonitis.[25] All these findings, along with changes observed in animal models of shock and sepsis, suggest that somatostatin merits further investigation as a mediator of pancreatic dysfunction in sepsis. However the widespread distribution of target cells and the limited number of receptor antagonists identified[26] will make such investigation difficult.

Endothelin, an endothelial-derived peptide with vasoactive properties, may have a role in the dysregulation of blood flow in sepsis. Evaluation of pancreatic blood flow with laser Doppler flowmetry in dogs revealed a reduction in blood flow after intravenous administration of endothelin.[27] Evidence for an important role of endothelin in microcirculatory disturbances in pancreatitis comes from experiments using endothelin receptor antagonists. This work has shown significant improvement in pancreatic microcirculation and a significant reduction in mortality rate in severe experimental pancreatitis.[28] The improvement in pancreatic blood flow was accompanied by improved urine output and stabilised capillary permeability.

Nitric oxide is thought to be among the pathophysiological factors contributing to disturbances in the pancreatic function in critical illness. The nitric oxide system is involved in pancreatic exocrine function,[29] as well as splanchnic perfusion.[14] The substrate for nitric oxide generation, L-arginine, and nitric oxide donors such as glyceryl trinitrate or sodium nitroprusside, attenuate the ischaemia-reperfusion injury in the pancreas and improve overall splanchnic flow.[29–31]

Recent animal studies have demonstrated that administration of lipopolysaccharide (LPS or endotoxin) induces expression of pro-inflammatory cytokines including tumour necrosis factor (TNFα), interleukin-1β (IL-1β) and IL-8 in acinar cells.[32] LPS challenges also induce expression of mRNA for pancreatitis-associated protein in the acinar cells, and at the same time reduces amylase mRNA levels. This suggests that in sepsis, pancreatic acinar cells may not only be subjected to microcirculatory changes, but may also be involved in the inflammatory response. Pancreatic dysfunction has similarly been reported in patients with sepsis.[33]

Pancreatic enzymes may themselves have a pivotal role in the activation of leucocytes and endothelial cells in shock. Such an action would have profound effects on microcirculatory flow profiles and the entire inflammatory response which ensues. In a study using homogenates from various rat organs (small intestine, spleen, heart, liver, adrenals, and pancreas) a dramatic increase in activation of naïve leucocytes was demonstrated only after incubation with pancreatic homogenates.[34]

Table 7.1 Ranson's eleven prognostic signs.[35]

On admission	Non-biliary pancreatitis	Biliary pancreatitis
Age (years)	>55	>70
Leucocytosis ($\times 10^9$)	>16	>18
Blood glucose (mmol/l)	>11·1	>12·2
Lactate dehydrogenase (IU/l)	>350	>400
Aspartate aminotransferase (IU/l)	>250	>250
After the first 48 hours		
Decrease in haematocrit (points)	>10	>10
Calcium (mmol/l)	<2	<2
Increase in blood urea nitrogen (mmol/l)	>1·8	>0·7
PaO_2 (mmHg)	<60	<60
Base deficit (mmol/l)	>4	>5
Fluid deficit (litres)	>6	>4

Each criterion has a value of 0 or 1. The Ranson's score is calculated by adding together all these values.

Grading the severity of the disease

For the last 20 years the Ranson criteria[35] has been the predominant score used to assess the severity and provide a mortality prediction. The Ranson score (Table 7.1) differentiates between biliary and non-biliary pancreatitis and relies on a proportion of contributory values being obtained after 48 hours. The cumulative score can then be used to calculate an estimated mortality (Table 7.2). Despite its widespread use, there are two major disadvantages of this score. Firstly a complete assessment cannot be made until 48 hours after admission or onset of acute pancreatitis. This is not particularly useful to clinicians who, at the time of admission need to be able to identify patients who warrant early and aggressive intervention in an attempt to improve outcome. Secondly the score lacks sensitivity in predicting outcome (Table 7.3). The same problems apply to the Glasgow

Score devised some ten years after Ranson by Blamey, Imrie and colleagues,[36] which although easier to use, still requires variables to be assessed at 48 hours.

Table 7.2 Ranson's prognostic criteria: mortality rate.

Number of positive criteria	Mortality rate
1 or 2	Less than 1%
3 or 4	15%
5 or more	40%

Each criterion has a value of 0 or 1. The Ranson's score is calculated by adding together all these values.

Table 7.3 Revised CT grading system for acute pancreatitis.[37,38]

Grade	Contrast-enhanced CT scan findings	CT severity index points	Morbidity %
A	Normal	0	0
B	Focal or diffuse pancreatic enlargement (changes restricted to pancreas)	1	0
C	Peripancreatic changes (without fluid collection)	2	7
D	Single extra pancreatic fluid collection	3	42
E	Two or more fluid collections or gas in or around the pancreas	4	60

In an attempt to improve the prognostic grading of severity of acute pancreatitis attention has turned to evaluating the potential of dynamic contrast-enhanced computed tomography (CT) scanning. CT provides the best means to visualize and diagnose pancreatitis and its local complications and may also be used for guiding percutaneous catheter drainage. In severe acute pancreatitis there is lack of normal enhancement with contrast of the entire gland or a portion thereof, which is consistent with pancreatic necrosis. Pancreatic necrosis is defined as diffuse or focal areas of non-viable parenchyma. Microscopically, there is evidence of damage to the parenchymal network, acinar cells and pancreatic ductal system and necrosis of perilobular fat. Areas of necrosis are often multifocal and rarely involve the whole gland. Necrosis develops early in the course of the disease and is usually well established by 96 hours after the onset of symptoms.[39]

The extent of pancreatic necrosis and the degree of peri-pancreatic inflammation has been used to determine outcome. Necrosis can be estimated as involving <30%, 30–50%, or >50% of the pancreatic gland, and categories A to E represent the spectrum of peri-pancreatic inflammation (see Table 7.3). The extent of necrosis and the grade of peri-pancreatic inflammation are combined to give a CT severity index, otherwise known as the Balthazar score (Table 7.4).[37] The score has been validated in terms of excellent correlation between the CT-depiction of necrosis and the development of complications and death (Table 7.5).[38]

Table 7.4 Relationship between CT grading system and morbidity.[37,38]

Necrosis	% Pancreas failing to enhance with intravenous contrast	CT severity index points	Morbidity %
None	None	0	12
Mild	0–30%	2	40
Moderate	30–50%	4	75
Extensive	>50%	6	100

Table 7.5 Relationship between total CT severity index points and morbidity.[37,38]

Total CT severity index points	Morbidity %
0–3	8
4–6	35
7–10	92

Current United Kingdom guidelines (1998) recommend a CT scan in severe acute pancreatitis between three and 10 days after admission and only earlier when the initial diagnosis is in doubt.[40] Enhanced prognostic information can be gained from the site of necrosis,[41] with involvement of the head of the pancreas being associated with a worse outcome.

However, the acceptance of CT as the gold standard in predicting poor outcome[42] has left the clinician with the age-old dilemma of how to identify on admission or within the early hours of the illness, those patients who would benefit most from critical care. It has been suggested that, practically, an admission acute physiological and chronic health evaluation (APACHE) II score of 8 or more and organ dysfunction involving at least one organ would be an acceptable predictor.[43–45] This combination in one study was associated with 55% mortality.[43]

Admission biochemical prognostic markers also exist. These include increased C-reactive protein, which is a good discriminator of mild and severe disease at 48 hours,[46] reduced serum selenium concentrations[47] or elevated plasma neutrophil elastase α_1-protease inhibitor concentrations.[48]

Additional markers include obesity (body mass index >30)[49] and left-sided or bilateral pleural effusions within 24 hours of admission[50] both of which predict poor outcome.

Pathophysiology of acute pancreatitis

The majority of cases of acute pancreatitis are mild and self-limiting. These usually resolve after a period of bowel rest, analgesia and fluid and electrolyte replacement. The remaining patients progress to acute severe pancreatitis, characterised by extensive pancreatic and retro-peritoneal inflammation, with superimposed patchy or generalised areas of necrosis and haemorrhage in the pancreas and surrounding tissues, and in some cases multiple organ dysfunction.

The clinical course of severe acute pancreatitis can be divided into a "toxaemic" early phase (0–15 days) characterized by the emergence of secondary organ dysfunction and the later "necrotic" phase when local complications occur. These phases may overlap, especially when infection occurs at an early stage.

Local complications

Infected pancreatic necrosis

Infected pancreatic necrosis is more common in biliary pancreatitis and is related to the degree of pancreatic necrosis, with 40–60% of patients developing infection. The infection usually originates from within the bowel itself and can significantly influence mortality. The peak occurrence time is around day 14, and 75% of such infections are caused by Gram negative organisms, with staphylococci and streptococci accounting for 20%. Anaerobic organisms account for only 10% of cultures. Other significant pathogens include fungi, which have had an increasing emergence over the last decade. The earlier the infection occurs, the higher the mortality, as early mixing of bacteria with ongoing enzymatic and necrotic processes appears to result in a highly toxaemic reaction and amplifies distant tissue injuries. In an attempt to reduce such infections there has been interest in both prophylactic antibiotic administration and selective gut decontamination.

Diagnosis of infection is supported by positive blood cultures and particularly by the presence of air bubbles in the retroperitoneum on abdominal CT scan. Percutaneous aspiration of pancreatic exudates guided by abdominal CT can reveal organisms on Gram stain or culture, which should lead to prompt surgical debridement.

Pseudocysts and abscesses

Pseudocysts develop in 10–20% of patients in the presence of severe acute pancreatitis; these are more common in alcoholic patients. Areas of necrosis may be too large to be absorbed and become sealed off by scarring, to form a cystic lesion (pseudocyst) filled with semi-solid debris, which liquefies and expands. This is a sterile process reflecting the activity of the digestive and lysosomal enzymes of pancreatic and leucocyte origin. The ducts in surviving functional areas of the pancreas may drain into pseudocysts so they may contain pancreatic enzymes in high concentrations. Pseudocysts vary in size from 1 to 30 cm in diameter. Large pseudocysts may rupture leading to pancreatopleural or pancreatopericardial fistulae, or more commonly, pancreatic ascites, resulting in chemical peritonitis. Alternatively, pseudocysts may cause compression and obstruction of the duodenum and/or the common bile duct. Rarely, a pseudocyst may extend to erode a major blood vessel, causing massive haemorrhage or leading to vascular thrombosis, manifesting as bleeding, perforation, fistulae, or late strictures.

Necrotic tissue presents a fertile medium for bacterial growth, and evolving pseudocysts may become infected by bacteria or fungi yielding a pancreatic abscess in 30–50% of cases. The micro-organisms may reach the pseudocyst by haematogenous or transmural routes. The absence or presence of micro-organisms distinguishes between pseudocysts and abscesses although abscesses and pseudocysts are otherwise generally similar macro- and microscopically. Over 50% of abscesses are polymicrobial with a predominance of enteric bacteria and *Candida albicans* is often cultured in patients previously treated with broad-spectrum antibiotics. Pancreatic abscesses usually occur when the active phase of pancreatitis is over; this often tends to be a more indolent process. Remote complications are less frequent; mortality is lower and sometimes a state of relative well-being interplays between the toxaemic phase and the clinical emergence of abdominal sepsis.

Remote organ dysfunction

The multiple organ dysfunction syndrome seen in severe acute pancreatitis is indistinguishable from that seen in the systemic inflammatory response syndrome (SIRS) or sepsis, and systemic complications contribute significantly to morbidity and mortality.

Toxic substances increase capillary permeability throughout the body and may reduce peripheral vascular tone, thereby intensifying hypotension. Circulating activated enzymes may damage tissues directly (for example phospholipase A2 is thought to injure alveolar membranes in the lungs).

The haemodynamic profile of the early phase is usually hyperdynamic, although severe myocardial depression may occur. Intravascular volume depletion due to increased vascular permeability, abdominal fluid sequestration and haemorrhage all play an important role, as well as a myocardial depressant factor released by acinar cells, and the release of prostenoids, PAF and cytokines by activated leucocytes in the necrotic areas.

Metabolic sequelae include an increase in resting energy expenditure (125% predicted), increased protein catabolism, unsuppressed hepatic gluconeogenesis and peripheral insulin resistance resulting in hyperglycaemia. Diabetic ketoacidosis or non-acidotic diabetic coma may be a presenting feature, particularly in patients with hyperlipidaemia.

All patients with severe acute pancreatitis develop pleural effusions, and 20% will develop acute respiratory distress syndrome (ARDS). Other complications include diaphragmatic splinting due to abdominal pain and/or ileus. This may lead to the development of secondary pulmonary atelectasis, hypoxaemia, and pulmonary infection.

Disseminated intravascular coagulation (DIC) is common and mostly results from the overwhelming inflammation cascade with activation of thrombotic and fibrinolytic pathways and, the proteolytic effects of circulating free trypsin.

Endothelial dysfunction and multiple organ dysfunction syndrome

Endothelial dysfunction is increasingly recognised as being of paramount importance in the ultimate development of multiple organ dysfunction syndrome or MODS. The role played by adhesion molecules in the evolution of dysfunction offers an opportunity for clinicians to target endothelial events. Such events may offer a more realistic time frame for intervention. Up-regulation of endothelial cell expression of the adhesion molecules, E-selectin and P-selectin, is important for endothelial/leucocyte interactions. Levels of serum soluble E-selectin and P-selectin have been suggested as markers of endothelial activation. A recent study demonstrated that during the first three days of admission, concentrations of serum soluble E-selectin increased in patients with severe acute pancreatitis while remaining relatively constant in patients with mild disease.[51] In contrast, concentrations of serum soluble P-selectin fell significantly during the first three days, with no significant difference between patients with mild or severe disease; however concentrations were significantly higher in non-survivors than survivors.[51]

Early enthusiasm for a PAF antagonist (Lexipafant)[52,53] has waned with the recognition that treatment was only effective if administered within the first 48 hours of the first symptoms. Other future strategies might include antibodies to the adhesion molecules, inter cellular adhesion molecule-1 (ICAM-1) and platelet endothelial cell adhesion molecule-1 (PECAM-1), the antioxidant N-acetylcysteine, which affects expression of a number of inflammatory responses including adherence, or the β_2 agonist dopexamine,[54] which has been shown to possess anti-inflammatory properties.[55]

Clinical relevance of cytokines

The initiating events leading to the development of necrosis are still poorly understood, although the role of cytokines, heterogeneous low molecular weight proteins with pleiotropic, redundant biological effects via highly specific receptors, have considerable importance in the pathophysiological process of severe acute pancreatitis.[56–59] Among the family of cytokines with predominantly pro-inflammatory effects, several experimental and clinical studies have shown that TNFα[60–62] and IL-1β[60,63–65] play a pivotal role in promoting local tissue destruction and remote organ failure in the course of the disease.

During experimental pancreatitis, upregulation of specific members of the IL-1 family of genes including IL-16 and its receptor antagonist (IL-1ra) occurs within the pancreatic parenchyma.[66] Such changes are indicative of pancreatitis severity and administration of IL-1ra attenuated pancreatitis severity and acinar cell necrosis, and improved survival in the animal model. In IL-1 receptor or IL-1 converting enzyme (ICE, caspase-1) gene-deleted ("knockout") mice, the lethality of experimental pancreatic injury was reduced by 70%.

In addition to IL-1, IL-18 is also cleaved into its active form by caspase-1. Circulating concentrations of IL-18 are significantly elevated in patients with acute pancreatitis complicated by necrosis and remote organ failure. These present data suggest an important role for caspase-1 dependent cytokine activation in the mechanism of severe acute pancreatitis beyond the experimental setting. In this context, IL-18 and/or caspase-1 may offer a potential target for new therapeutic approaches.[67]

Controversies in Management

Prophylactic antibiotics

Randomised controlled clinical trials have previously failed to show any benefit from prophylactic antibiotic administration in acute pancreatitis.[68–70] However, these studies had serious flaws. Firstly, the studies included patients with mild pancreatitis, in whom an infection of the pancreas is a rarity. Secondly, these studies used antibiotics which we now know do not penetrate the pancreas. Thirdly the antibiotics used do not adequately cover the spectrum of bacteria that are normally found in severe acute pancreatitis. Newer clinical trials taking into account the problems of previous studies indicate a benefit of antibiotic therapy in the prevention of infection.[71] In Italy, Pederzoli et al. randomized 74 patients with mild, moderate and severe pancreatitis in an open, multi-centre, clinical trial. Patients were randomised within 72 hours of onset to receive imipenem or no antibiotic.[72] The incidence of pancreatic infection was significantly reduced in the treated group (12·2% versus 30·3%, $p < 0.01$), and there was a trend towards decreased mortality. More recently Bassi *et al.* compared imipenem with perfloxacin in 60 patients with severe necrotising pancreatitis ($>50\%$ necrosis).[73] Although fluoroquinolones should theoretically offer excellent protection against infection of necrosis, the incidence of infected necrosis was significantly higher than among the patients receiving imipenem (infected necrosis 34% versus 10%, extrapancreatic infection 44% versus 20%, $p < 0.05$). Mortality was not significantly affected. Given the available evidence, both carbapenems or broad-spectrum third generation cephalosporins seem to be valid options.[74] These antibiotics should penetrate into the pancreatic gland and adjacent fatty tissue and should cover the bacteria most commonly identified.[75] As yet there are no studies available to determine the appropriate duration of treatment.

Selective decontamination of the digestive tract

A transperitoneal route for translocation of bacteria, leading to infection of the inflamed pancreas and peripancreatic tissue has been demonstrated in rats.[76] In controlled trials of selective decontamination of the digestive tract (SDD) the incidence of Gram negative pancreatic infection was significantly reduced in treated patients.[77] Mortality was also reduced (22%) compared to untreated patients (35%). However, the use of SDD has been reported to be associated with the emergence of resistant *Staphylococcus aureus* and an increased incidence of ventilator-acquired pneumonia. It is likely that this and the inconvenience of administering SDD are the reasons why this therapy has not been widely adopted.

Enteral or parenteral nutrition in acute pancreatitis

Patients with severe acute pancreatitis face increasing metabolic demands throughout the course of the disease,[78] and hence the provision of nutritional input is an essential part of supportive therapy. Failure to prevent malnutrition, leading to a prolonged negative nitrogen balance, increases mortality rates. The advocates of enteral nutrition have, by and large, won the debate regarding the route of feeding.[79] However, the site of enteral feeding – pre or post ligament of Trietz, the composition of the enteral nutrition, and when to commence feeding – remain a topic of discussion.

It is fair to state that the importance of tube positioning has not been evaluated but our personal opinion is that the tube should be placed distal to the third part of the duodenum, thereby avoiding superimposed stimulation of the pancreas by cholecystokinin. The choice of feed is more controversial especially in cases where there is little or no necrosis. In this population there currently exist a number of immunomodulating feeds, which contain novel substrates such as arginine, short chain fatty acids, glutamine and added supplements, including a combination of antioxidants (see *Critical Care Focus Volume 7: Nutritional Issues*[80]). There is an increasing body of evidence that suggests these feeds may have the propensity to alter beneficially immune function, and the inflammatory process.[81,82] In the presence of extensive necrosis a pre-digested feed becomes mandatory.

Antioxidants

Antioxidant therapy has been advocated to combat the "oxidative stress" of acute pancreatitis. It is not feasible, except in specific medical conditions, to prevent the burst of free radical activity within pancreatic acinar cells. Clinical experience suggests that early administration of parenteral antioxidants may prevent the downward spiral towards haemorrhagic pancreatic necrosis and multiple organ failure, provided the chosen agents can enter the pancreatic acinar cells. Experimental evidence and antioxidant profiles in admission blood samples strongly suggest that a combination of ascorbic acid (vitamin C), selenium, methionine, N-acetylcysteine, β carotene, and tocopherol (vitamin E) will be beneficial. Clinical trials are currently underway and should provide evidence for future therapy.

Controversial pharmacological agents

Anti-secretory strategies remain controversial in the acute setting. Somatostatin and its long acting analogue octreotide are potent inhibitors of pancreatic secretion. Both agents also stimulate reticuloendothelial system activity and play a regulatory role, mostly inhibitory, in the modulation of the immune response. To date several small studies have shown benefit with octreotide in patients with severe acute pancreatitis, with reference to septic complications and development of ARDS, circulatory failure, and mortality.[83] Large scale randomized trials are now awaited and it is prudent to await their outcome before adopting therapy bearing in mind that octreotide is a potent vasoconstrictor of the splanchnic circulation.

Clinical Intervention

Endoscopic retrograde cholangiography

Endoscopic retrograde cholangiography (ERCP) is only indicated when a biliary cause is strongly suspected or, preferably, proven. A previous history of a typical biliary colic is helpful in this respect. Sonographically detected gallstones and/or dilated biliary ducts and jaundice strongly support a biliary origin. An alanine aminotransferase activity above 80 IU/L is very specific for biliary pancreatitis but only 50% sensitive and isolated mild hyperbilirubinaemia is a non-specific sign.[84]

Trials of ERCP differ importantly with regard to inclusion criteria, study design and definitions[85–88] and therefore definite conclusions about timing are not possible. However, recommendations are provided in the 1998 United Kingdom guidelines for the management of acute pancreatitis.[40] In the presence of severe pancreatitis with sonographically detected gallstones and jaundice (or a bilirubin level equal or greater than twice the upper level of normal) or aspartate or alanine transaminase activity at least twice the upper limit of normal, or in the case of cholangitis, urgent ERCP with sphincterotomy is recommended. In the absence of these biochemical findings and clinical signs a conservative treatment is justified in suspected gallstone pancreatitis. However, if the patient's condition fails to improve within 48 hours in spite of intensive resuscitation, an experienced endoscopist should carry out therapeutic ERCP and the patient should receive antibiotic coverage.

Surgical treatment

The timing and type of surgical intervention for patients with acute necrotising pancreatitis remains controversial.[89,90] Infected necrosis is generally accepted as an absolute indication for aggressive surgical debridement and surgery should be performed as soon as possible after confirmation of pancreatic infection. However, available evidence does not support a general operative policy towards patients with sterile necrosis although subgroups may benefit from surgical intervention. Such subgroups include patients with multiple organ failure who continue to deteriorate despite full intensive care; patients continuing to exhibit an infective picture 10 days or more after onset; patients with recurrent abdominal pain or hyperamylasaemia following attempts at oral feeding three to four weeks after onset. Others however, believe surgery is unnecessary as long as the necrotic process remains sterile.[91]

Due to the local inflammatory process the intra-abdominal pressure can rise leading to a fall in cardiac output, elevated central venous pressure and pulmonary capillary wedge pressure, elevated peak airway pressure and oliguria as a consequence.[92] It has been suggested that if the intra-abdominal pressure exceeds 20 to 25 mmHg a decompressive laparotomy may be necessary. The most widely used technique to estimate the intra-abdominal pressure involves transurethral measurement of urinary bladder pressure using a Foley catheter.

Conclusion

Acute pancreatitis is an inflammatory disease characterised by wide clinical variation and ruled by its complications. Pancreatitis occurs fairly frequently in critically ill patients, as a result of pancreatic ischaemia and reperfusion or circulatory factors and clinicians must be vigilant of the mechanisms which lead to such pancreatic dysfunction. Irrespective of the aetiology of the pancreatitis the main determinant of outcome remains the site and extent of pancreatic necrosis. The early use of contrast-enhanced CT will identify the population with the greatest mortality and such patients should receive early and aggressive critical care management. In the presence of pancreatic necrosis, prophylactic antibiotic therapy should be instituted with an antibiotic which can achieve a bactericidal concentration within the pancreatic tissue, such as imipenem or ceftazidime. Antibiotic therapy should be adjusted in the light of positive results from regular fine needle pancreatic aspirations. Attention should also be paid to early feeding, preferably using the jejunal enteral route, and strategies should be employed to preserve the splanchnic microcirculation. At present there is insufficient evidence to recommend the routine use of octreotide. and pancreatic surgery should be reserved only for the treatment of infected pancreatic necrosis, or late complications, such as a pseudocyst.

Hopefully in time potential new targets for therapeutic intervention will emerge.

References

1   Braganza JM, Scott P, Bilton D, et al. Evidence for early oxidative stress in acute pancreatitis. Int J Pancreatol 1995;17:69–81.
2   Steer ML, Meldolesi J. Pathogenesis of acute pancreatitis. Annu Rev Med 1988;39:95–108.
3   Anderson RJL, Braganza JM, Case RM. Routes of protein secretion in the isolated cat pancreas. Pancreas 1990;5:394–400.
4   Case RM. Secretory polarity. In Braganza JM, ed, The Pathogenesis of Pancreatitis. Manchester UK: Manchester University Press, 1991, 34–44.
5   Arvan P, Castle JD. Phasic release of newly synthesised secretory proteins in the unstimulated rat exocrine pancreas. J Cell Biol 1987;104:243–52.
6   Rinderknecht H. Acute necrotising pancreatitis and its complications: an excessive reaction of natural defence mechanisms? In Braganza JM, ed, The Pathogenesis of Pancreatitis. Manchester UK: Manchester University Press, 1991, 86–100.
7   Tran DD, Cueta MA, Schneider AJ, Wesdorp RIC. Prevalence and prediction of multiple organ system failure and mortality in acute pancreatitis. J Crit Care 1993;8:145–53.
8   Fernandez-Cruz L, Navarro S, Valderrama R, et al. Acute Necrotising Pancreatitis: A multi-centre study. Hepato-Gastroenterology 1994;41:185–9.
9   Menger MD, Bonkhoff H, Vollmar B. Ischaemia-reperfusion-induced pancreatic microvascular injury. An intravital fluorescence microscopic study in rats. Dig Dis Sci 1996;41:823–30.
10 Krejci V, Hiltebrand L, Banic A, Erni D, Wheatly Am, Sigurdsson GH. Continuous measurements of microcirculatory blood flow in gastrointestinal organs during acute haemorrhage. Br J Anaesth 2000;84:468–75.

11 Reilly PM, Toung TJ, Miyachi M, Schiller HJ, Bulkley GB. Haemodynamics of pancreatic ischaemia in cardiogenic shock in pigs. *Gastoenterology* 1997;**113**: 938–45.

12 Fish RE, Lang CH, Spitzer JA. Regional blood flow during continuous low-dose endotoxin infusion. *Circ Shock* 1986;**18**:267–75.

13 Fantini GA, Shiono S, Bal BS, Shires GT. Adrenergic mechanisms contribute to alterations in regional perfusion during normotensive E.coli bacteremia. *J Trauma* 1989;**29**:1252–7.

14 Booke M, Hinder F, McGuire R, Traber LD, Traber DL. Nitric oxide synthase inhibition versus norepinephrine in ovine sepsis: effects on regional blood flow. *Shock* 1996;**5**:362–70.

15 Raper RF, Sibbald WJ, Hobson I, Rutledge FS. Effect of PGE1 on altered distribution of regional blood flow in hyperdynamic sepsis. *Chest* 1991;**100**: 1703–11.

16 Hiltebrand LB, Krejci V, Banic A, Erni D, Wheatley AM, Sigurdsson GH. Dynamic study of the distribution of microcirculatory blood flow in multiple splanchnic organs in septic shock. *Crit Care Med* 2000;**28**:3233–41.

17 Kahle M, Lippert J, Willemer S, Pabst W, Martin P. Effects of positive end expiratory pressure (PEEP) ventilation on the exocrine pancreas in mini pigs. *Res Exp Med* (Berl) 1991;**191**:309–25.

18 Gullo L, Caviicchi L, Tomassetti P, Spagnolo C, Freyrie A, D'Addato M. Effects of ischaemia on the human pancreas. *Gastroenterology* 1994;**111**:1033–8.

19 Fernandez-del Castillo C, Harringer W, Warshaw AL, *et al.* Risk factors for pancreatic cellular injury after cardiopulmonary bypass. *N Engl J Med* 1991; **325**:382–7.

20 Harris AG. Somatostatin and somatostatin analogues: pharmacokinetics and pharmacodynamic effects. *Gut* 1994;**35(Suppl)**:S1–S4.

21 Revhaug A, Lygren I, Lundgren TI, *et al.* Release of gastrointestinal hormones in cardiodepressive shock. *Acta Anaesthesiol Scand* 1985;**29**:371–4.

22 Revhaug A, Lygren I, Lundgren TI, Jorde R, Burhol PG, Giercksky KE. Changes in plasma levels of gastrointestinal regulatory peptides during hemorrhagic shock in pigs. *Acta Chir Scand* 1985;**151**:401–7.

23 Revhaug A, Lygren I, Lundgren TI, Jorde R, Burhol PG, Giercksky KE. Release of gastrointestinal peptides during E.coli endotoxaemia. *Acta Chir Scand* 1984; **150**:535–9.

24 Briard N, Rico-Gomez M, Guillaume V, *et al.* Hypothalamic mediated action of free fatty acid on growth hormone secretion in sheep. *Endocrinology* 1998;**139**: 4811–19.

25 Almdahl SM, Osterud B, Melby K, Giercksky KE. Mononuclear phagocyte thromboplastin, bacterial counts and endotoxin levels in experimental endogenous gram-negative sepsis. *Acta Chir Scand* 1986;**152**:351–5.

26 Patel YC. Somatostatin and its receptor family. *Front Neuroendocrinol* 1999;**20**:157–98.

27 Takaori K, Inoue K, Kogire M, *et al.* Effects of endothelin on microcirculation of the pancreas. *Life Sci* 1992;**51**:614–22.

28 Foitzik T, Eibl G, Hotz HG, Faulhaber J, Kirchengast M, Buhr HJ. Endothelin receptor blockade in severe acute pancreatitis leads to systemic enhancement of microcirculation, stabilization of capillary permeability and improved survival rates. *Surgery* 2000;**128**:399–407.

29 Konturek JW, Hengst K, Kulesza E, Gabryelewicz A, Konturek SJ, Domschke W. Role of endogenous nitric oxide in the control of exocrine and endocrine pancreatic secretion in humans. *Gut* 1997;**40**:86–91.

30 Benz S, Schnabel R, Weber H, *et al.* The nitric oxide donor sodium nitroprusside is protective in ischaemia/reperfusion injury in the pancreas. *Transplantation* 1998;**66**:994–9.

31 Vollmar B, Janata J, Yamauchi JI, Menger MD. Attenuation of microvascular reperfusion injury in rat pancreas transplantation by L-arginine. *Transplantation* 1999;**67**:950–5.

32 Vaccaro MI, Calvo EL, Suburo AM, Sordelli DO, Lanosa G, Iovanna JL. Lipopolysacharide directly affects pancreatic acinar cells. *Dig Dis Sci* 2000;**45**:915–26.

33 Tribl B, Madl C, Mazal PR, *et al.* Exocrine pancreatic function in critically ill patients: septic shock versus non-septic patients. *Crit Care Med* 2000;**28**:1393–8.

34 Kistler EB, Hugli TE, Schmid-Schonbein GW. The pancreas as a source of cardiovascular cell activating factors. *Microcirculation* 2000;**7**:183–92.

35 Ranson JHC, Rifkind KM, Roses DF, *et al.* Prognostic signs and the role of operative management in acute pancreatitis. *Surg Gynaecol Obstet* 1974;**139**:69–81.

36 Blamey S, Imrie C, O'Neill J, Gilmour W, Carter D. Prognostic factors in acute pancreatitis. *Gut* 1984;**24**:1340–6.

37 Balthazar E, Freeny P, van Sonnenberg E. Imaging and intervention in acute pancreatitis. *Radiology* 1994;**193**:297–306.

38 Balthazar E, Robinson D, Megibow A, *et al.* Acute pancreatitis: Value of CT in establishing prognosis. *Radiology* 1990;**174**:331–6.

39 Isenmann R, Buchler M, Uhl W, *et al.* Pancreatic necrosis: An early finding in severe acute pancreatitis. *Pancreas* 1993;**8**:358–61.

40 United Kingdom guidelines for management of acute pancreatitis. *Gut* 1998;**42** **(Suppl 2)**:S1–S13.

41 Kemppainen E, Sainio V, Haapianen L, *et al.* Early localization of necrosis by contrast-enhanced computer tomography can predict outcome in severe acute pancreatitis. *Br J Surg* 1996;**83**:924–9.

42 Bradley E III. A clinically based classification system for acute pancreatitis; summary of the international symposium on acute pancreatitis. *Arch Surg* 1993;**128**:586–90.

43 Bank S. Risk factors in acute pancreatitis – towards a classification based on clinical criteria. In: Gyr KE, Singer MV, Sarles H, eds. *Pancreatitis: concepts and classification.* Amsterdam: Excerta Medica, 1984, 389–94.

44 De Sanctis JT, Lee MJ, Gazelle GS. Prognostic indicators in Acute Pancreatitis: CT v APACHE II. *Clin Radiol* 1997;**52**:842–8.

45 Tenner S, Sica G, Hughes M, *et al.* Relationship of necrosis to organ failure in severe acute pancreatitis. *Gastroenterology* 1997;**113**:899–903.

46 Gudgeon A, Heath D, Hurley P *et al.* Trypsinogen activation peptides assay in the early prediction of acute pancreatitis. *Lancet* 1990;**335**:4–8.

47 Kuklinski B, Buchner M, Schweder R, *et al.* Akute pankreatitis – Eine 'Free Radical Disease' Letalitatssenkung Durch Natrium selenit (Na_2SeO_3) Therapie. *Z Gesame Inn Med* 1991;**5**:7–11.

48 Dominguez-Munoz JE, Carballo F, Garcia MJ. Monitoring of serum proteinase-antiproteinase balance and systemic inflammatory response in prognostic evaluation of acute pancreatitis. *Dig Dis Sci* 1993;**38**:507–13.

49 Suazo-Barahona J, Carmona-Sanchez R, Robles-Diaz G, *et al.* Obesity: a risk factor for severe acute biliary and alcoholic pancreatitis. *Am J Gastroenterol* 1998;**93**:1324–8.

50 Talamini G, Uomo G, Pezzilli R, *et al.* Serum creatinine and chest radiographs in the early assessment of acute pancreatitis. *Am J Surg* 1999;**177**:7–14.

51 Powell JJ, Siriwardena AK, Fearon KCH, Ross JA. Endothelial-derived selectins in the development of organ dysfunction in acute pancreatitis. *Crit Care Med* 2001;**29**:567–72.

52 Kingsworth AN. Early treatment with lexipafant, a platelet activating factor antagonist in human acute pancreatitis. *Gastroenterology* 1997;**112**:A453.

53 Abu-Zidan F. Hope or hype for lexipafant? *Nature* 1998;**395**:431.

54 Schmidt W, Hacker A, Gebhard MM, *et al*. Dopexamine attenuates endotoxin-induced microcirculatory changes in rat mesentery: Role of Beta-2 adrenoreceptors. *Crit Care Med* 1998;**10**:1639–46.

55 Byers RJ, Eddleston JM, Pearson RC, *et al*. Dopexamine reduces the incidence of acute inflammation in the gut mucosa after abdominal surgery in high-risk patients. *Crit Care Med* 1999;**27**:1787–93.

56 Formela LJ, Galloway SW, Kingsnorth AN. Inflamatory mediators in acute pancreatitis. *Br J Surg* 1995;**82**:6–13.

57 Kusske AM, Rongione AJ, Reber HA. Cytokines and acute pancreatitis. *Gastroenterology* 1996;**110**:639–42.

58 Norman J. The role of cytokines in the pathogenesis of acute pancreatitis. *Am J Surg* 1998;**175**:76–83.

59 Mayer J, Rau B, Gansauge F, *et al*. Local and systemic cytokines in human acute pancreatitis: Clinical and pathophysiological implications. *Gut* 2000;**47**:546–52.

60 Denham W, Yang J, Fink G, *et al*. Gene targeting demonstrates additive detrimental effects of interleukin-1 and tumour necrosis factor during pancreatitis. *Gastroenterology* 1997;**113**:1741–6.

61 Grewal HP, Mohey el Din A, Gaber L, *et al*. Amelioration of the physiological and biochemical changes of acute pancreatitis using an anti-TNF-α polyclonal antibody. *Am J Surg* 1994;**167**:214–19.

62 Hughes CB, Grewal HP, Gaber LW, *et al*. Anti TNF therapy improves survival and ameliorates the pathophysiological sequelae in acute pancreatitis in the rat. *Am J Surg* 1996;**171**:274–80.

63 Tanaka N, Murata A, Uda K, *et al*. Interleukin-1 receptor antagonist modifies the changes in vital organs induced by acute pancreatitis in a rat experimental model. *Crit Care Med* 1995;**23**:901–8.

64 Norman JG, Franz MG, Fink GS, *et al*. Decreased mortality of severe acute pancreatitis after proximal cytokine blockade. *Ann Surg* 1995;**221**:625–34.

65 Fink GW, Morman JG. Intrapancreatic interleukin-1β gene expression by specific leukocyte populations during acute pancreatitis. *J Surg Res* 1996;**63**:369–73.

66 Norman J, Yang J, Fink G, *et al*. Severity and mortality of experimental pancreatitis are dependent on interleukin-1 converting enzyme (ICE). *J Interferon Cytokine Res* 1997;**1**:113–18.

67 Rau B, Baumgart K, Paszkowski AS, Mayer JM, Berger HG. Clinical relevance of caspase-1 activated cytokines in acute pancreatitis: High correlation of serum interleukin -18 with pancreatic necrosis and systemic complications. *Crit Care Med* 2001;**29**:1556–62.

68 Howes R, Zuidema GD, Cameron JL. Evaluation of prophylactic antibiotics in acute pancreatitis. *J Surg Res* 1975;**18**:197–200.

69 Finch WT, Sawyers JL, Schenker S. A prospective study to determine the efficacy of antibiotics in acute pancreatitis. *Ann Surg* 1976;**183**:667–71.

70 Trudel JL, Thompson AG, Brown RA. Prophylactic use of antibiotics in pancreatic sepsis: 25-year appraisal. *Can J Surg* 1984;**27**:567–70.

71 Golub R, Siddiqi F, Pohl D. Role of antibiotics in acute pancreatitis: A meta-analysis. *J Gastrointest Surg* 1998;**2**:496–503.

72 Pederzoli P, Bassi C, Vesentini S, Campedelli. A randomised multicenter clinical trial of antibiotic prophylaxis of septic complications in acute necrotising pancreatitis with imipenem. *Surg Gynecol Obst* 1993;**176**:480–3.

73 Bassi C, Falconi M, Talamini G, *et al*. Controlled clinical trial of perfloxacin versus imipenem in severe acute pancreatitis. *Gastroenterology* 1998;**115**:1513–17.

74 Sainio V, Kemppainen E, Puolakkainen P, *et al*. Early antibiotic treatment in acute necrotising pancreatitis. *Lancet* 1995;**346**:663–7.

75 Buechler MW, Malfertheiner P, Friess H, *et al*. Human pancreatic tissue concentration of bacteriocidal antibiotics. *Gastroenterology* 1992;**103**:1902–8.

76 Medich DS, Lee TK, Melham MF, *et al*. Pathogenesis of pancreatic sepsis. *Am J Surg* 1993;**165**:46–50.

77 Luiten EJT, Hop WCJ, Lange JF, *et al*. Controlled clinical trial of selective decontamination for the treatment of severe acute pancreatitis. *Ann Surg* 1995;**222**:57–65.

78 Marulenda S, Kirby DF. Nutritional support in pancreatitis. *Nutrition Clin Prac* 1995;**10**:45–53.

79 Kalfarentos F, Kehagias J, Mead N, *et al*. Enteral nutrition is superior to parenteral nutrition in severe acute pancreatitis: results of a randomised prospective trial. *Br J Surg* 1997;**84**:1665–9.

80 Galley HF, ed. *Critical Care Focus Volume 7: Nutritional Issues*. London: BMJ Books/Intensive Care Society, 2001.

81 Gadek JE, De Michele SJ, Karlstad MD, *et al*. Effect of enteral feeding with eicosapentaenoic acid, gamma linolenic acid, and antioxidants in patients with acute respiratory distress syndrome. Enteral Nutrition in ARDS study group. *Crit Care Med* 1999;**27**:1409–20.

82 Wyncoll D, Beale R. Immunologically enhanced enteral nutrition; current status. *Curr Opin Crit Care* 2001;**7**:128–32.

83 Fielder F, Jauerig G, Keim V, *et al*. Octreotide treatment in patients with necrotising pancreatitis and pulmonary failure. *Intensive Care Med* 1996;**22**: 909–15.

84 Tenner S, Dubner H, Steinberg W. Predicting gallstone pancreatitis with laboratory parameters: a meta-analysis. *Am J Gastroenterol* 1994;**89**:1863–6.

85 Neoptolemos J, Carr-Locke D, London N, Bailey I, James D, Fossard D. Controlled trial of urgent endoscopic retrograde cholangio pancreatography and endoscopic sphincterotomy versus conservative treatment for acute pancreatitis due to gallstones. *Lancet* 1998;**2**:979–83.

86 Fan S, Lai E, Mok F, Lo C, Zheng S, Wong J. Early treatment of acute biliary pancreatitis by endoscopic papillotomy. *N Engl J Med* 1993;**328**:228–32.

87 Nowak A, Nowakowska-Dulawa E, Marek T, Rybicka J. Final results of the prospective, randomised, controlled study on the endoscopic sphincterotomy versus conventional management in acute biliary pancreatitis. *Gastroenterology* 1995;**108 (Suppl A)**:380 (abstract).

88 Fölsch U, Nitsche R, Lüdtke R, *et al*. Early ERCP and papillotomy compared with conservative treatment for acute biliary pancreatitis. *N Engl J Med* 1997; **336**:237–42.

89 Poston G, Williamson R. Surgical management of acute pancreatitis. *Br J Surg* 1990;**77**:5–12.

90 Farthmann E, Lausen M, Schoffel U. Indications for surgical treatment of acute pancreatitis. *Hepatogastroenterology* 1993;**40**:556–62.

91 Dervenis C, Johnson C, Bassi C, *et al*. Diagnosis, objective assessment of severity and management of acute pancreatitis. *Int J Pancreatol* 1999;**25**:195–210.

92 Nathens A, Boulanger B. The abdominal compartment syndrome. *Curr Opin Crit Care* 1998;**4**:116–20.

Index

Page numbers in **bold** type refer to figures; those in *italic* refer to tables or boxed material.